The Complete Guide to
Ocular History
Taking

Janice K. Ledford, COMT
EyeWrite Productions

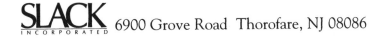 6900 Grove Road Thorofare, NJ 08086

The Complete Guide to
Ocular History Taking

Janice K. Ledford, COMT
EyeWrite Productions

SLACK
INCORPORATED
6900 Grove Road Thorofare, NJ 08086

www.slackbooks.com

ISBN: 978-1-55642-369-7

Copyright © 1999 by SLACK Incorporated

Published by: SLACK Incorporated
                 6900 Grove Road
                 Thorofare, NJ 08086-9447 USA
                 Telephone: 856-848-1000
                 Fax: 856-853-5991
                 www.slackbooks.com

Contact SLACK Incorporated for more information about other books in this field or about the availability of our books from distributors outside the United States.

Ledford, Janice K.
The complete guide to ocular history taking / Janice K. Ledford
    p. cm.
Includes bibliographical references and index.
ISBN 1-55642-369-1 (alk. paper)
1. Eye—Diseases—Diagnosis. 2. Medical history taking.
3. Opthalmic assistants. I. Title.
[DNLM: 1. Eye Diseases—diagnosis. 2. Medical History Taking.
WW 141L473c 1998]
RE79.H57L43 1998
617.7'15—dc21
DNLM/DLC
for Library of Congress   98-36725
                                                             CIP

Printed in the United States of America.

Last digit is print number: 10 9 8 7 6 5 4 3 2

Dedication

This book is dedicated to Virginia Cole Veal: artist, poet, mentor, aunt, and dear friend.

Table of Contents

Acknowledgments

This page is always one of my favorite to write. Putting someone's name in print as a means of thanking him or her falls way short of the wonderful things he or she deserves. If I could, I'd put each name in neon lights and flash it across the sky.

First, thank you so much to Charles G. Kirby, MD, for his editorial assistance. He patiently waded through pages and pages of history questions and never got tired of telling me that "pain" is a good word. ("Dolor, dolor," he cried in red letters on my manuscript copy. I wanted to couch it and say "discomfort," but, as he reminded me, pain and discomfort are two different things.) I also appreciate his kindness and courtesy as we work together in the clinic each week.

I gave Tom Turrentine, OD, the nickname of "Coding King" because of his understanding of the HCFA regulations and coding guidelines. His help was essential to getting Chapter 1 in shape.

Since completing his Physician Assistant degree in 1994, I have had to start thanking Jim Ledford for his medical assistance as well as husbandly support. "Medical assistance" refers not only to reviewing the manuscript and answering innumerable medical questions, but also to keeping me healthy. (He's gotten very good at treating the *disease du jour*). I would have no writing career at all if it weren't for his ability (and willingness) to cheerfully endure.

There are others who deserve to be mentioned as well: Todd Hostetter, COMT (for information and leads on HCFA regulations); the staff of Western North Carolina Eye Care Associates; Ronnie Massey, MD (for medical information and opinion); G. Henry Wall, RPh (for information on currently available ophthalmic drugs); and Mark Friedman, Product Manager of PDR, Medical Economics (for data regarding the PDR).

Over the years, the staff of the Book Division at SLACK Incorporated have moved from the category of work acquaintances to friends. It's almost to the point where I'm afraid to name names because so many people do such a great job in order to keep books coming for ophthalmic and optometric personnel. While I want to say thanks to you all, I must specifically mention John Bond, Amy Drummond, and Debra Christy.

Finally, thanks to my boys, who are getting used to the idea that their mom is a writer. Every book, article, or story that comes out with my name on it is also a tribute to their patience and tolerance of what I do for a living. It's easy to excuse Mom from being there when she's away working in the eye clinic. But it's harder to understand when she's just upstairs "playing on her computer." TJ, I'm glad you finally got a vehicle of your own. Thanks for the "road work" you now do for me. Collin, I hope you enjoy having my "old" computer in your room. Thanks for all the times that you fed the cat. And thank you both for helping me learn how to navigate on the Internet. I couldna' done it without ya!

About the Author

This is the sixth SLACK book to bear the name Janice K. Ledford, COMT, as an author. Jan wandered into ophthalmology in 1982 after obtaining a degree as a dental hygienist. Within 6 years, she worked her way through the certification levels to become an ophthalmic medical technologist. In addition to clinical duties, she's functioned as instructor, continuing education coordinator, and staff writer in the several eye clinics where she has been employed. She now works part-time for the Western North Carolina Eye Care Associates.

In 1985, Jan began developing her second career, that of a medical writer. She started her own company, EyeWrite Productions, for the purpose of writing and editing medical materials, primarily in ophthalmology. In addition to the SLACK books, she is the co-author of an eye-care book for laymen, *The Crystal Clear Guide to Sight for Life* by Starburst Publishing. Jan is also the Series Editor for SLACK's *Basic Bookshelf for Eyecare Professionals*. Her articles have appeared in *Ophthalmology*, *Ophthalmology World News*, *Annals of Ophthalmology and Glaucoma*, *Contact Lens Spectrum*, and the *Journal of Ophthalmic Nursing and Technology*, among others.

Jan's writing talents are not limited to the medical field and non-fiction, however. She is an award-winning fiction writer whose novel, *Hannah*, was released by Guideposts Books in October 1997. She is a member of the National League of American Pen Women.

Jan and her husband, Jim, reside in the mountains of western North Carolina with their two teenage boys (TJ and Collin) and four cats. She enjoys good friends, good books, and good music. She plays handbells in the church choir and bowls with her husband on a Monday night league. She does not like snakes.

Foreword

As a general ophthalmologist practicing for more than 30 years, I am daily made more aware of the importance of a well-done preliminary patient work-up by an ophthalmic technician. The quality of my exam is largely dependent upon the information furnished by the technician.

Ophthalmology is a most beautiful and exciting endeavor when there is precision supported by accurate data. As in all disciplines of medicine, an intelligent history is the foundation of the patient work-up. With the complexity of medicine today and the increased need for documentation, a manual devoted to ophthalmic history taking is a welcome addition to the ophthalmic literature. No one is more eminently qualified on this subject than Jan Ledford, COMT, a nationally acclaimed writer on ophthalmic technology. In her usual lucid and concise style, she takes the reader through the maze of the ophthalmic history, mapping out a blueprint for a thorough and useful document.

This book fills a valuable niche in ophthalmology and will be much appreciated by everyone in the field, whether a novice technician, resident, or veteran clinician. Jan Ledford also labors in the trenches of clinical ophthalmology, drawing from the patient the same nuggets of information she details in this exciting new book. Read on, learn, and enjoy!

—Charles G. Kirby, MD
WNC Eye Care Associates

Introduction

In the early 1990s, the Joint Commission on Allied Health Personnel in Ophthalmology (JCAHPO) conducted a survey of tasks performed by certified ophthalmic medical personnel (OMPs). More than 1,500 physician employers responded to the survey. They were asked to rate the importance of 77 different tasks commonly performed by OMPs in their practices, universities, and clinics. The number one most important task, according to these ophthalmologists, was history taking.

To visualize the importance of the history, think of the times that the patient in your exam chair was a pre-verbal child, an aphasic adult, or a non-English-speaking senior. Most likely, these patients were accompanied by someone who could tell you the history or interpret for the patient. But suppose that there was no advocate for them. Without being able to ask the patient any questions, you'd have to find out what was wrong based only on objective findings. And there would be other problems. For example, the physician wouldn't have any idea whether or not the patient might be allergic to the medication that could solve the problem. The history is used to find out what is bothering the patient, as well as to glean background information pertinent to any possible treatment, recurrence, or complications.

More recently, the history (and the thoroughness thereof) has become an issue in fair billing practices. While our first concern is good patient care, the Health Care Financing Administration (HCFA) has issued guidelines regarding elements of the examination as they relate to coding (and, subsequently, billing). This has added a new dimension to the task of "taking a history."

History taking is, thus, one of the most critical tasks delegated to OMPs. If it is too scanty or incomplete, the physician must pick up the slack and take the time to further question the patient. He or she must do this for two reasons. First, proper information is needed before diagnosis and treatment can be rendered. Second, the coding guidelines must be satisfied (however, this application walks a precarious line). In the interest of efficiency, it is obviously to everyone's advantage for the OMP to take a proficient history to begin with. That's what this book is all about.

History taking is a skill like any other; it must be studied, then practiced. Unlike other parts of the exam, the ocular history is not a once-and-done type of task; it begins when you call the patient back to the exam room (or even before that, if you have the patient's previous records in hand). But the potential for adding to the history doesn't end until you complete all your testing and walk out the exam room door.

The goal of this book is to teach you the basics of ocular history taking. In many cases, the text gives you actual questions to ask the patient that depend on the patient's needs, problems, and potential diagnoses. While my desire was to be thorough, you may find that the questions given here are much more detailed than suits your purpose (or time constraints) on a day-to-day basis. However, such details are often the key that turns the lock to diagnosis and treatment. Thus, I realize that you are faced with a dilemma: what information is actually important? There can be only one answer: any information that your physician/employer thinks is important. Now and then, every OMP should spend time in the exam room while the physician is with a patient. Listen for the "extra" questions (beyond those recorded in your history) that he or she asks the patient. Next time, ask the patient these questions yourself. If you don't understand the rationale behind the questions, ask the doctor later (outside the exam room). Learning why a question is important will help you become a better history taker.

There is another dimension of history taking worth mentioning. Your attention to the patient during the interview process plays a key role in rapport and the patient's sense of satisfaction with the visit. As Mark Twain noted, everyone has a story to tell. We might well add that most everyone wants to tell that story. The history gives them that opportunity.

An ophthalmologist friend of mine is fond of saying, "Listen to the patient, and he'll tell you what's wrong." What else is this task of listening but history taking? Good interviewing is a combination of public relations and medical knowledge. It is my hope that this book will help you develop skills in both.

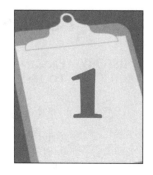

How to Take an Ophthalmic History

The primary purpose of the history is to gather pertinent information that will help the physician diagnose and treat the patient.

History Taking and Coding

The history or, more accurately, the depth of the history also plays a key role in coding. Coding refers to a determination of the level of the patient's exam (Table 1-1). The three key components for determining the level of service for each patient visit are history, examination, and medical decision making. Other minor items that come into play are counseling, coordination of care, nature of presenting problem, time, and medical necessity.[1]

The higher the level of service (as determined by the codes), the higher the billing rate. For example, a complete eye exam on a new patient is of a different level than a pressure check on a returning glaucoma patient with no other problems. There is also a difference if the returning glaucoma patient needs only a pressure check or if, while there, he or she also states that his or her vision has been blurry. In the first case, the code is for a simple, uncomplicated (ie, "problem focused") exam. In the second case, the patient needs more, starting with a more complete history of present illness and perhaps a review of certain systems. That will probably be followed by lensometry,

Table 1-1
Elements of history affecting exam level.*

HISTORY	PROBLEM FOCUSED	EXPANDED PROBLEM FOCUSED	DETAILED	COMPREHENSIVE
	CC Brief HPI (1-3 elements)	CC Brief HPI (1-3 elements)	CC Extended HPI (4+ elements or status of at least 3 chronic or inactive conditions)	CC Extended HPI (4+ elements or status of at least 3 chronic or inactive conditions)
	No ROS	Problem pertinent ROS (1 system)	Extended ROS (2-9 systems)	Complete ROS (10+ systems)
	No PFSH	No PFSH	Problem Pertinent PFSH (1 element)	Complete PFSH (3/3 elements)

CC: chief complaint   ROS: review of systems
HPI: history of present illness   PFSH: past, family, and social history
from the American Medical Association

refractometry, and, perhaps, ophthalmoscopy. Plus, the physician's professional judgment as to what is causing the blurriness is required (in addition to judging whether or not the intraocular pressure is acceptable and whether or not the patient needs an adjustment in glaucoma medications). This second exam is more complicated and gets a code with a higher billing rate, and justifiably so.

Of course, it's unethical (and illegal) to "do more" during the examination and treatment just to be able to bill at a higher rate. There has to be a reason to "do more." That reason must be documented in the history in the form of a patient complaint. Then, the tests we do are justified. We are supposed to document what occurred during the patient's visit and code from there; we are not supposed to document in order to meet a specific service level.

To make sure that we don't bill higher (or lower) than the exam warrants, the Health Care Financing Administration (HCFA) has issued guidelines about these coding and billing matters. These guidelines are causing some major panic in health care as we all scramble to learn how to work with the system, because "violators will be prosecuted." As of this writing, however, no one knows exactly when the guidelines will be finalized.

While all this coding and billing is not the sole responsibility of ancillary personnel, we must be aware of what's going on in order to assist our employers with compliance. As far as the history goes, certain elements (discussed later) must be present for the exam to qualify for a specific level of coding. These requirements will no doubt change periodically, so you need to check with your employer and/or office manager for the current criteria.

Important note: It is not the intention of this book to advise you on the coding guidelines or how to interpret and meet them. This book is written solely as an aid to thorough patient care. Coding is mentioned because it is a fact of life you must be aware of, and to leave it out would compromise the completeness of this text. To learn about coding, check the appropriate references at the end of this book or visit the HCFA website at www.HCFA.gov.

Patient Confidentiality

Anything that the patient tells you during history taking must be treated as confidential information. We sometimes ask questions regarding private details of the patient's life (such as drug-abuse issues). In addition, some patients are more sensitive than others about sharing any information (such as their age). The patient has the right to refuse to answer a question or to refuse to talk to anyone but the physician about the matter.

A patient who balks over sharing a piece of information may decide to divulge the answer after hearing your reason for asking a specific question. The patient who asks to speak only to the doctor can be cheerfully reassured that you have no problem with that. But, you might also say, "Dr. Soper has asked me to do some preliminary testing for her before she sees you. It will help me know which tests she'll need if you don't mind giving me an idea of the type of problem you might be having. Anything you tell me is held in strictest confidence." This may be all that is needed to prompt the patient to permit the history. If he or she still refuses, you have no choice but to inform the physician and move on.

Whether you verbally "promise not to tell" or not, all patient information must be kept strictly confidential. You may not discuss the patient's history, test results, or other medical information with anyone not directly involved in his or her care unless the patient has given express permission. You may, for example, take the chart to your supervisor and ask for advice on what tests to run if you're not sure. You may not, however, go to the employee lounge and say, "Hey, did you see that lady in the pink dress? She's been in alcohol rehab 10 times in the past 3 years!" In cases where the need to discuss the patient's history with others is bona fide, make sure you do so out of the hearing of any other person.

What if the patient has brought a relative or friend along? If you don't know who's who, look at the chart and ask, "Which of you is Mrs. Collins?" When the patient identifies herself, you might then ask, "Do you want your friend to come into the exam room with you?" This gives the patient the option to say yes or no, relieving you of the responsibility of a third person hearing the patient's history (albeit known to the patient). Most patients who bring someone with them do so out of a need for moral support or, in some cases, for an interpreter.

Rapport and Interview Skills

History taking starts before you call the patient back. If the patient is new, glance over the information sheet(s). If the patient is a follow-up or a returning annual exam, review the last exam, but don't write anything down yet. You've got to verify everything with the patient before writing it down.

The history serves a secondary function, which is also important. It gives you the opportunity to establish rapport with the patient. So when you call the patient back to do the history, smile! If it's a patient you've never helped before, introduce yourself. Say, "Mrs. Meeks, my name is Margaret, and I'm an optometric/ophthalmic assistant. I'll be working with you a little bit today before Dr. Soper sees you." Then, help the patient get comfortable. Seat yourself at eye level with and facing the patient.

Starting off with a brief bit of "small talk" may set the tone for the exam and help relax the patient. Because you've already reviewed the patient information, perhaps you can comment from that. Something that you might have in common is best. ("I see that you live on Victor Drive. I grew up two blocks from there! Did you ever buy apples from that little produce stand on the corner?") Even a comment about the weather will work.

When you start the history, don't ask questions with your head buried in the chart. Yes, you have to make notes, but you can make some eye contact as well. (You might tell the patient, "I'll be making some notes as we talk.") Use body language that says you're interested. This patient is the most important person in your world—at least for this particular moment. Lean forward in your chair a little (but not too close—stay out of his or her "personal space"). These nonverbal indicators go a long way toward building rapport. You can also use comments that show your ongoing interest (such as "Yes" and "I see.") To the patient, it's not so much a matter of how long you (or the doctor) spend with him or her, it's whether or not you were really there while you were there.

Touching the patient in an effort to create rapport has become controversial. Offering to shake the patient's hand during introductions is generally acceptable. Other touching may be perceived by the patient as comforting or friendly—or as threatening or sexual. The nurturing side of most of us involved in health care makes us sensitive to the fact that the only caring touch the patient might receive that entire day (or week, or month) came from us during an office visit. However, today's litigious society makes us hesitant to offer such contact. If your employer has a policy on physical contact with patients, follow it. If you have no policy, at least discuss the matter. Use discretion and common sense.

I mentioned that you must verify everything on the patient information sheet. On the other hand, I think it's rude to ask the patient to take the time to fill out the form, then repeat the questions in the exam. I've had patients get irritated and say, "I answered that on the form!" So here's a possible solution. Pull the sheets apart, so the patient can see that you're referring to the form he or she filled out. Say, "Mrs. Cole, thanks for filling this form out. Let me verify this information while I transfer it into your formal medical record of today's exam." If the patient is returning for an annual exam, you could say, "Mrs. Taylor, let me update the information you gave us last time you were here. I see that your mother has diabetes. Has anyone else in the family developed diabetes in the past year?"

Sometimes, the history becomes a tug-of-war between the patient and the technician. The patient does not run the history—you do. You've got to be in control; otherwise, your history will take 30 minutes. I was taught, like you were, that it is rude to interrupt someone, especially someone older. But I've learned over the years that patients don't seem to mind being interrupted— they don't usually even notice. You are the detective here; you are the one trained in eye care; you have the best notion of what the doctor needs to know. The patient realizes that he or she is there for an eye exam and won't mind tactful interruptions when you steer the conversation back on track with specific questions about vision and/or eyes.

So, do your best to keep the patient on track. If she starts talking about her garden club, interrupt her and bring her back to the eye exam. If she says, "I was about to tell you that," say, "I'm sorry. Go ahead. You said your eyes watered when you were playing bridge?" You've been nice, but you've still re-directed the conversation.

As the history progresses, take a little extra effort to let the patient know that he or she is getting through to you. You might use the technique of echoing some of the patient's words. For example, the patient states, "I had general anesthesia to have some teeth cut out and after I woke up, I found that I couldn't see to read up close anymore. I had to hold the paper way out in front of me so I could see it." You could say, "You had to hold the paper out?" Echoing comments like this lets the patient know you are listening, interested, and concerned. As this example points out, however, history taking is not the time to correct any misconceptions that the patient has about vision and/or the eyes. That can be handled later, perhaps when the physician is discussing the diagnosis.

Finally, once you have all the details on the patient's presenting complaint (discussed in a moment), give the patient a summary of what you think you've heard. "Mrs. Aleshire, let me repeat this back to you now, to be sure I've got it right." These interview and communication skills, combined with common sense and good manners, will ensure that your history is complete, accurate, and builds good will.

Questions, Questions

Questions are the tools of history taking. To keep the interview moving and on target, the questions should be well-chosen. Several different types of questions may be appropriate. First, there are the general, broad questions that are useful when getting started. These are nondirective questions, or questions that do not ask about specifics, but are designed to get the ball rolling. An example: "Are you having any problems with your eyes?" Directive questions are used to begin to fill in the details and are directed at getting specific information, for instance, "You said that your vision is doubled?" Finally, you might use closed or forced-choice questions, which require short, specific answers, such as, "Is your vision blurred all day, or does it come and go?"

Sometimes, you may have to rephrase a question if the patient doesn't understand (or if you suspect he or she doesn't understand). And don't forget to watch your language! Use terms that the patient can understand. Instead of asking, "Is the redness inferior to the iris?" you should ask, "Is it red underneath the colored part of your eye?" This is not the time to show off your knowledge of medical terminology.

If the patient has difficulty telling you when a particular problem started, you might offer some choices in order to pinpoint the details you need. You might say, "Has it been bothering you a few days? A couple weeks? For months?" Or, you might prompt him or her by using holidays: "Did it bother you before Christmas?"

Avoid asking combination questions. If you ask the patient, "Is your eye red, or does it hurt?" and the patient says, "Yes," how are you going to know which question the patient is answering? Give the patient a chance to answer one question before asking another.

The History and Protocol

The history should be governed by protocol—in other words, done pretty much the same way every time. This helps ensure that you won't forget an item. HCFA has dictated the elements of an ophthalmic history as pertains to coding (Table 1-2 and 1-3). These elements are the chief complaint (CC); history of present illness (HPI); review of systems (ROS); and past, family, and/or social history (PFSH).

Your office may use a cookbook style exam form that prompts you to follow a certain order, which is fine. Such forms also make coding easier. We will discuss each part of the history here. Chapter 2 gives more details as to specific questions to ask.

Table 1-2
Elements of the history affecting exam level*

CODE/ COMPONENT	99211	99212	99213	99214	99215
NATURE OF PRESENTING PROBLEM	Minimal severity	Self-limited or minor severity	Low to moderate severity	Moderate to high severity	Moderate to high severity
HISTORY	Evaluation and management code does not require the presence of a physician	**PROBLEM FOCUSED** CC Brief HPI (1-3 elements)	**EXPANDED PROBLEM** Focused CC Brief HPI (1-3 elements)	**DETAILED** CC Extended HPI or status of at least 3 chronic or inactive conditions)	**COMPREHENSIVE** CC Extended HPI (4+ elements or status of at least 3 chronic or inactive conditions)
		No ROS	Problem pertinent ROS (1 system)	Extended ROS (2-9 systems)	Complete ROS (10+ systems)
		No PFSH	No PFSH	Problem pertinent PFSH (1 element)	Complete PFSH (2/3 elements)

*from the American Medical Association

Chief Complaint (CC)

In general, it is common to start off by eliciting the CC. The CC is the main problem for which the patient has come in. Ask, "Are you having any particular problems with your eyes?" Then listen. Don't write yet, unless it's just to make a few notes. The patient may give three or four problems. Often, the problems will be in a recognizable "cluster," such as floaters and flashes. If the problems seem unrelated, ask, "Which one of those bothers you the most?" and start playing detective with that. Then, you can go back and catch the other problems one at a time.

What do you do about the patient who says, "No problems, it's just time for my check up?" First, commend them for keeping up with their eye care. Then go fishing. I understand that if the patient is on Medicare, there must be a complaint or the company won't pay for the exam. While you cannot force a CC from the patient, you can ask questions designed to elicit a CC if one

Table 1-3
Elements of the history*

CHIEF COMPLAINT   NOTE: ROUTINE EYE EXAMINATIONS NOT COVERED

HISTORY OF THE PRESENT ILLNESS (HPI)	ELEMENTS	LEVEL
	Location	Brief = 1-3 elements
	Quality	Extended = 4 or more elements
	Severity	
	Duration	
	Timing	
	Context	
	Modifying factors	
	Associated signs & symptoms	
	or	
	Status of at least 3 chronic or Inactive illnesses	

REVIEW OF SYSTEMS (ROS)	SYSTEMS	LEVEL
	Constitutional	Problem pertinent = 1 system
	Eyes	Extended = 2 to 9 systems
	Ears, nose, mouth, throat	Complete = 10+ system
	Cardiovascular	
	Respiratory	
	Gastrointestinal	
	Genitourinary	
	Musculoskeletal	
	Integumentary (skin and/or breast)	
	Neurological	
	Psychiatric	
	Endocrine	
	Hematologic/lymphatic	
	Allergic/immunologic	

PAST, FAMILY, SOCIAL, HISTORY (PFSH)	ELEMENTS	LEVEL
	Past history	Pertinent = 1 element
	Family history	Complete = 2 or 3 elements[†]
	Social history	3 elements required: new outpatient visits, consultations (outpatient & initial inpatient)

[†]2 elements required: establish patients
*from the American Medical Association

exists. You might start by looking at the patient's past record, if he or she has been in before. See what problems he or she was having before. "Mrs. James, when you were here last year, your eyelids were itching. Are you still having a problem with that?" Also, check the last diagnosis, and formulate questions from that. Suppose Mrs. James had nuclear sclerosis at the last visit. You could ask if she's experienced any problem with glare, halos around lights at night, problems with depth perception, or any number of symptoms that a person with cataracts might have. That way you might hit on a complaint.

If that method doesn't work, start asking about vision. "Do you feel like your glasses are doing the job? Can you still see road signs? Are you having any problems seeing to read?" If that still doesn't produce a CC, ask if his or her glasses are holding up all right. Are the lenses scratched? Has he or she thought about trying a progressive (no-line) lens?

Regardless of the patient, "no complaints" alone is not an adequate history, ever. However, there will be occasional patients who honestly have no complaints. Remember our glaucoma patient returning for an intraocular pressure (IOP) check? She has no complaints. You write: "Patient states she has glaucoma and is here for an IOP check. Vision seems stable. States excellent compliance with meds." While this may not be very helpful from a coding perspective, it is good patient care. Coding is not the be-all, end-all of medicine. Taking care of patients is.

History of Present Illness

Once you have a CC, you need more information about it. There are eight elements that make up the history of present illness (HPI). Documenting information about one to three of them constitutes a brief exam. If there are four or more elements present in the history, then the service is considered extended. (This may change; keep current with HCFA rules.)

Here are the eight elements along with sample questions to illustrate their meanings:

1. Location—Which eye is bothering you? Where does it hurt?
2. Quality—Describe the pain. Is it dull or stabbing? Constant? Throbbing?
3. Severity—On a scale of 1 to 10, how bad is the pain?
4. Duration—How long has it been going on? Did it come suddenly or gradually?
5. Timing—Does it occur all the time or just sometimes? When? For how long?
6. Context—What were you doing when this started?
7. Modifying factors—What seems to make it better or worse? What have you tried to correct the problem? Did that help?
8. Associated signs and symptoms—Do other symptoms or problems occur along with this? (For example, light flashes followed by a headache or light flashes accompanied by floaters.)

Sometimes, a patient will come in with a CC that has a long duration. Suppose it's a new patient who complains of fluctuating vision. When you ask how long it's been going on, she says, "Oh, maybe 3 or 4 years." So you ask if she's been seen for that problem before, and she says, "no." This leaves you scratching your head. Your first thought might be to say, "Why haven't you seen about it until now?" but that sounds judgmental, and perhaps a little rude. (I suppose it depends a lot on the tone of your voice.) But you'll get more useful information if you ask, "Has something about the problem changed that made you come to see about it now?"

Some questions will come to you as you learn more and gain experience. Certain symptoms will suggest other questions that you need to ask. For example, suppose the patient complains of light flashes. Retinal detachment (RD) and posterior vitreous detachment (PVD) can cause this. So, in addition to the eight types of questions above, you should also ask about other symptoms of RD and PVD: Have you noticed any floaters? Has the vision gotten dimmer? Has the vision blacked out? Do you seem to have a curtain over part of your vision? Suppose that the patient responds, "No," to all of these. Light flashes could possibly be migraine headaches, so you ask, "Describe the flashing. How long does it last? Do you have a headache after that?" History taking really is detective work. You have to consider what might be causing the symptoms and ask other appropriate questions.

Once you've gathered all the information regarding the CC, ask the patient, "Why do you think that your eyes are blurry, itching, etc.?" Recording the patient's thoughts may help the physician.

Review of Systems

When I started in the eye care field in 1982, we didn't get into a lot of depth beyond asking if the patient had hypertension or diabetes. Now, with Medicare rules, we have had to expand our questioning a lot. Plus, patients have come to expect more all-encompassing care from specialists.

The portion of the history known as review of systems (ROS) may overlap the past medical history (covered in the next section). During the ROS, you ask the patient about different parts of his or her body. (Specific questions are given in Chapter 2.) Often these questions are phrased as symptom-related. For instance, instead of asking about heart conditions, you would ask if the patient ever experienced chest pain.

To avoid getting a lot of trivial details about various minor complaints and past problems, you might try using the word "serious" when you ask your patients these questions. For example, "Mrs. Aleshire, have you had any serious problems with your muscles or joints?" You do want to know if she has osteoarthritis; you don't want to hear about the ache in her left elbow that occurs once or twice a year.

Past, Family, and Social History (Standard Database)

It's time to shift gears. We've been talking about the presenting problem, but that's not all there is to a history. Now we move on to establishing the background history, or what some call the standard database. The standard database establishes the patient's background health information, old problems, co-existing minor problems, medications, social history, family history, and ROS. Any of these items may contain information that will affect the diagnosis and treatment for that patient.

Past Medical History

I generally like to ask about the patient's medical history first, followed by the medications. The medical history will include items such as hospitalizations, surgeries, injuries, illnesses, pregnancy, and childbirth. For each "Yes," you'll have to get more information, such as year of occurrence or onset. This is also the time and place to record the patient's last visit to both the regular doctor and eye doctor.

Sometimes, the patient's systemic problems will prompt more history questions. Diabetes is a good example. Even if a diabetic has no visual complaints, you need to know how long he or she has been diabetic and how it's treated. "Mrs. Parrish, is your sugar level stable? Has it been stable for the past 6 or 8 weeks? How often do you have it checked? What does it usually run? Do you notice any change in your vision when it runs high or low?" (For specific questions related to specific systemic problems, see Chapter 4.)

The patient's medicines should more or less coordinate with his or her medical problems. If the patient is taking Lopressor (Geigy Pharmaceuticals, Summit, NJ), but denies having hypertension, you should double-check things. The patient may have misunderstood the original question. Now and then, a patient will say, "I don't have high blood pressure because I'm taking medicine that keeps it normal." And sometimes a patient is taking a medication for a nonstandard reason. For example, Inderal (Wyeth-Ayerst Laboratories, Philadelphia) is usually given for hypertension, but some patients take it for migraine headaches.

Another reason you must not automatically transfer information from the patient information sheet onto the chart without verifying it is that patients are often poor spellers. They may also misunderstand what they are taking. Suppose the patient tells you he or she is taking Zantax. There is no such medication. There is Zantac (Glaxo Pharmaceuticals, Research Triangle Park, NC), and there is Xanax (The UpJohn Company, Kalamazoo, MI). The first is for stomach ulcers and reflux, the second is nerve medication. So you must ask the patient, "Is that for your stomach or for your nerves?"

Assistants can be poor spellers too, but when in doubt look it up (see Chapter 3 or Appendix B). When patients don't know what they are taking, ask whom their medical doctor is or where they get their prescriptions filled. Then call. Have the pharmacist spell the names for you as you enter them in the chart.

If the patient brings in a paper bag with medicines in it, you still have to ask about them. Just because it's in the bag doesn't mean he or she is taking it. Just because the Timoptic (Merck and Co., Inc, West Point, PA) bottle is labeled twice a day doesn't mean she's using it twice a day. You've got to ask.

Insulin injections are always recorded by type and dose. You can even do it as a chart, listing what type of insulin is taken, when, and how much.

On eye medications, you must record the name and the dosing schedule.

If it's a medication that comes in different strengths and types, such as pilocarpine, you'll need to write down the strength as well. For glaucoma medicines, write down the last time the patient used it.

You will often have to ask specifically if the patient takes any over-the-counter (OTC) medication regularly. They think that OTC medicine doesn't count. But suppose the patient is taking vitamin A and doesn't tell you, then the physician puts him or her on vitamin therapy for macular degeneration, which includes high amounts of A. Now the patient may be overdosing on vitamin A, but no one knows it. Other items that patients often forget include patches, monthly hormone or allergy shots, and aspirin.

Next, ask about drug allergies. You should also make a note as to how that drug affected the patient. There is a difference between a true allergy and a side effect. Itching, rash, and shortness of breath are allergies. Nausea and vomiting are probably side effects. In addition, note any drugs that the patient's doctor has told him or her not to take. For example, a patient who is already on blood thinners may have been told not to take aspirin, as it would further thin the blood.

Family History

When taking the family history, you are looking for serious illnesses and major conditions among the patient's blood relatives. (If a patient mistakenly tells you about his or her spouse, it may be best just to ignore the information rather than remind him or her that the spouse is not a blood relative.) In eye care, we are most interested to know if there is a family history of glaucoma, cataracts, macular degeneration, strabismus, amblyopia, and other such major problems. Systemically, we are most interested in hypertension and diabetes. But you should also ask, "Are there any other health problems that run in your family?" Even here, a positive response can lead to other questions you should ask. If the patient doesn't have diabetes, but there is a positive family history, you should ask, "When was the last time you had your blood sugar tested?" The same could apply to any other positive finding.

Social History

The social history can be difficult to ask for, because it is so personal. You need to know about the patient's current life and any habits that may affect his or her health. Here again, the wording of the questions can make all the difference. Instead of asking, "Do you smoke? Do you drink?" it is better to ask, "Do you use tobacco products? Do you use alcohol?" If the patient answers, "Yes," say, "Tell me about that." Instead of asking about drug abuse, ask "Have you ever used recreational drugs?" Also, instead of asking someone (especially an elderly woman) if he or she lives alone, ask if he or she lives with someone. If not, ask if there is someone nearby who looks in on him or her now and then. (And don't assume that just because an adult is single that he or she lives alone!)

The patient's occupation and hobbies are very important in the ophthalmic history, because we must make sure that visual correction will be adequate at the distances needed. In addition to the "whats," you should also ask such things as whether or not eye protection is worn and the distance to work surfaces.

Before you finally move from history taking into the physical exam, give the patient one more chance. Always ask, "Is there anything else about your health or your eyes that you think Dr. Conrad needs to know?"

Other History Notations

You may need to make a few notes in the chart that stem from your personal observations of the patient during the history. For example, suppose the patient complains that he or she "can't see a thing" after a work-related injury, yet he or she walked into the exam room without assistance. While this is not exactly history taking, it is important information and should be noted in the record.

It is sometimes pertinent to make a note regarding the patient's psychological demeanor on the day of the exam. A patient who knows what day it is and where he or she is at the moment is generally considered to be oriented.

We spoke earlier about how your attitude toward the patient is conveyed through eye contact and posture. The patient's nonverbal communication can also indicate his or her state of mind. The patient who leans toward you is indicating her interest and involvement. The patient who leans away from you may be telling you that you are too close, or may be conveying his or her desire to escape the situation. Tightly crossed arms and legs may indicate defensiveness or tension. Other signs of tension include clenching the fists, drumming the fingers, fidgeting, and talking fast. Avoiding eye contact may signal that the patient is shy, ashamed, submissive, or deceptive. Speaking slowly in a low tone of voice may indicate sadness. The angry patient may speak in a higher pitch at first, then in a lower pitch as he or she attempts to control his or her emotions. A change from "negative" signals to "positive" ones during the history may indicate that you've been successful in building rapport with this patient. Any severe reaction indicated by the patient's body language should be noted.

In addition, a comment about the patient's affect (state of mind) or reaction to you and the history taking process may be warranted. A patient with a normal affect may still seem a little nervous about the exam, but will smile and maybe laugh when appropriate. A flat affect refers to a general lack of emotion on the part of the patient. An inappropriate affect refers to an emotional reaction that is out of harmony with the situation. Finally, a labile affect means that the patient displays rapid shifts in emotional state. These types of observations may be extremely important, especially if the patient is being considered for surgery.

Because of the sensitive nature of psychological issues and the fact that OMPs are not usually trained in psychology, it may be best to record such comments on a sticky note for the physician. He or she can then decide if it needs to be a permanent part of the patient's record.

Also, make a note about anything personal the patient tells you that might be good for the physician to know. This could include the name that the patient prefers to go by or the fact that today is his or her birthday, anniversary, etc. The patient may share some personal achievement, and the physician will want to extend congratulations. If a spouse or other family member has recently died, the doctor will appreciate knowing this as well.

Documentation

Your history should begin with the day's date, the patient's name, and identifying information (patient's age, sex, and race). If there is more than one person doing histories, you should initial your entry.

When eliciting the CC, first listen to the patient, then condense the narrative on the exam sheet. Some physicians and practices want the history to be recorded from your point of view. That is, you are an impartial person who is recording another person's story. Other offices prefer that the history be a paraphrase of the patient's own words. In the first case, you would note, "Patient complains of a pressure sensation behind both eyes." In the second case, you would write, "Patient states, 'It feels like something is pushing from behind my eyes'."

It is important to note that a negative response should be recorded if you asked about an entity that the patient does not have. This is especially pertinent when going through the review of systems (explained earlier). If you ask the patient, "Have you ever had any serious problems with your heart?" and the patient says, "No," then you should record "none" in the chart as a note on the cardiovascular system. This proves that you did ask. (And also shows why so many practices are using pre-printed exam forms.)

If you have to correct or change something in the entry, you should draw one single line through that material and initial the change. Don't totally scratch it out, and never use White-Out™ or erase anything. This goes for any correction in the chart.

Documentation is also the key to coding and billing. This is true for the entire exam, of course, and that includes the history. As one physician notes, "In the past, a code was determined by work done. Documentation had to do with patient care, not with coding and reimbursement levels. This is no longer the case. Today, coding and reimbursement are determined by documentation, not the work done. So, if it isn't written down, it didn't happen, it can't be used to calculate the code and it can't be billed."[2] We might add that if it's not legible, it's not written down.

Anatomic Landmarks

The use of anatomic landmarks and directions can be very helpful in condensing and documenting the narrative (Figures 1-1 through 1-3c).

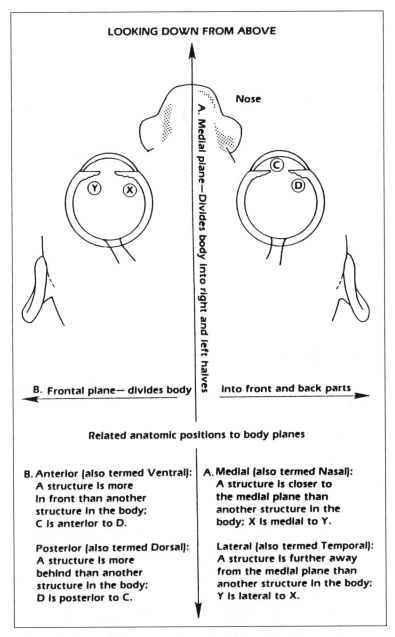

LOOKING DOWN FROM ABOVE

Nose

A. Medial plane—Divides body into right and left halves

B. Frontal plane— divides body | Into front and back parts

Related anatomic positions to body planes

B. Anterior (also termed Ventral):
A structure is more
in front than another
structure in the body;
C is anterior to D.

Posterior (also termed Dorsal):
A structure is more
behind than another
structure in the body;
D is posterior to C.

A. Medial (also termed Nasal):
A structure is closer to
the medial plane than
another structure in the
body; X is medial to Y.

Lateral (also termed Temporal):
A structure is further away
from the medial plane than
another structure in the body;
Y is lateral to X.

Figure 1-1 Anatomical directions (reprinted with permission from Nemeth SC, Shea CA. *Medical Sciences for the Ophthalmic Assistant.* Thorofare, NJ: SLACK Incorporated; 1988).

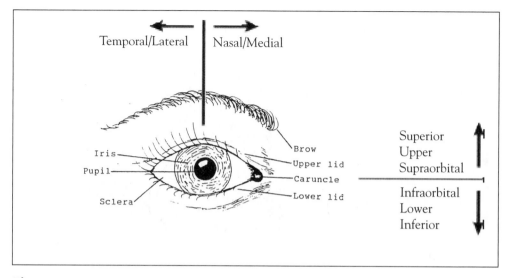

Figure 1-2 Anatomical directions of the eye (drawing by Holly Hess. Adapted from *The Crystal Clear Guide to Sight for Life,* Starburst Publishers. Reprinted with permission).

Giving Reassurance and Advice

Sometimes, the patient is rather distraught while giving the history. He or she may have been experiencing the problem for a long time and may be worried about going blind. Because you are identified as medical personnel, the patient may ask you, "What do you think is wrong?" or "Do you think anything can be done for this?"

Of course, it is not the role or responsibility of auxiliary personnel to give the patient a diagnosis. It is usually best to tell the patient, "Well, we really haven't done all the testing we need yet. Once Dr. Foss sees you, we'll know more."

It is also important to never say anything to a patient (or the patient's spouse, parents, or other caregivers) that sounds like a guarantee that medical treatment will cure something. For example, it would be unwise to tell the patient, "Oh, Dr. Foss will put you on some drops that will clear your eye right up!" You've attempted to encourage the patient, but there may be things about the patient's eye condition that you don't know. Such "guarantees" are especially dangerous if the patient has experienced trauma or is considering a surgical procedure. Never tell any patient that "everything will be all right." If it doesn't turn out "all right," you may have to eat your words—in court. But it is acceptable to offer nondescript reassurance such as, "I know that Dr. Foss will do everything he can for you."

It is also beyond the realm of the eye care paraprofessional to give the patient advice. You should tell the patient, "Dr. James will explain what he

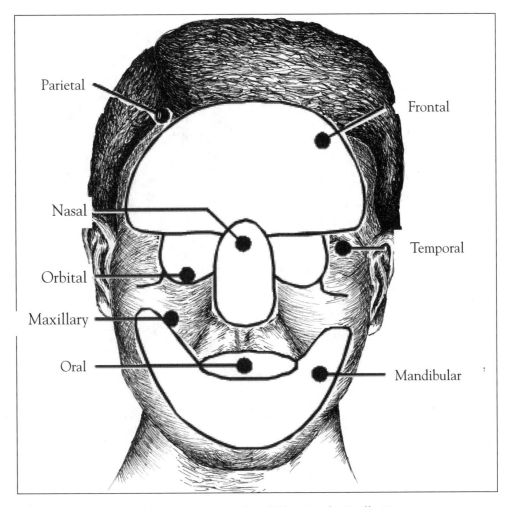

Figure 1-3a Anatomical locations on the head (drawing by Holly Hess).

wants you to do after he's examined you."

In some situations, however, it may be appropriate to share information. For example, suppose the patient is a 38-year-old man who complains that he's having trouble seeing up close. He asks you, "Don't people usually need reading glasses around age 40?" It would be sensible to briefly explain presbyopia. But you may want to follow the explanation with a statement such as, "Of course, we won't know if that's what is affecting you until Dr. Rogers sees you. After she's examined you, she'll explain everything."

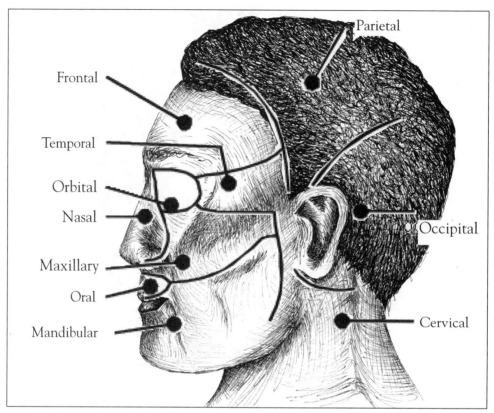

Figure 1-3b Anatomical locations on the head (drawing by Holly Hess).

A Final Note

Probably the key word for history taking is patience. We've all had patients like this:

You: Mrs. Jones, are you taking any medications?

Mrs. Jones: No.

As you write down "none," she suddenly continues:

Mrs. Jones: Except for Lasix (Hoechst-Roussel Phramaceuticals, Inc., Somerville, NJ)and potassium and Estratest (Solvay Pharmaceuticals, Inc., Marietta, GA).

You scratch through "none" and record her list. Then she continues:

Mrs. Jones: Well, the doctor took me off the Estratest at my last visit....

And so it goes. Just keep your sense of humor, and remember that what you're doing really does make a difference.

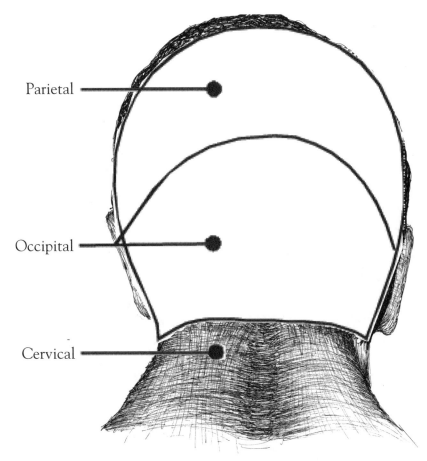

Parietal

Occipital

Cervical

Figure 1-3c Anatomical locations on the head (drawing by Holly Hess).

References

1. *Documentation in Depth: A Comprehensive Guide for Physicians.* St. Paul, MN: Medical Learning, Inc.; 1997.
2. Gayton JL, Bittinger MD. How we fixed our coding problem. *Ophthalmology Management.* 1998;24(1):26-29.

Basic History Questions

This chapter lists specific questions to ask the patient during the routine history-taking process. The first part of the text covers the normal eye exam; you will notice that the subheadings are the actual history elements. The second section of the chapter deals with specific types of exams (such as contact lenses, strabismus, etc.) as well as specific patient populations (including the pregnant, pediatric, and geriatric patient).

The Routine Eye Exam

Chief Complaint (History of Present Illness)

- Are you having any particular problems with your eyes? Or, What brings you to the eye doctor today?

Note: Then see Chapter 5 for questions regarding specific symptoms.

- What other problems do you have with your eyes?
- Which one of those bothers you the most?
- Do you feel like your glasses are doing the job? Can you still see road signs? Are you having any problems seeing to read?
- Has something about the problem changed that made you come to see about it now?

For each complaint, you must investigate further by asking the following types of questions:

1. Location—Anatomically or directionally, where the problem occurs (for example, in the right eye or the left side of the vision).
2. Quality—Describe the problem in detail (for example, pain is sharp or dull; vision is doubled or blurry).
3. Severity—On a scale of 1 to 10, how bad is _____ ?
4. Duration—How long has this been going on? Did this come on suddenly or gradually?
5. Timing—Does it occur all the time or just sometimes? When? For how long?
6. Context—What were you doing when this started?
7. Modifying factors—What seems to make it better? Worse? What have you tried to correct the problem? Did that help?
8. Associated signs and symptoms—Do other symptoms or problems occur along with this? (For example, light flashes followed by a headache or light flashes accompanied by floaters.)

Background History (Standard Database)

Past Medical History
- Have you had any type of surgery? What? When? Were there any problems afterward, such as uncontrolled bleeding?
- Have you had any serious illnesses? What? When? Were you hospitalized?
- Have you had any serious injuries? What? When? Were you hospitalized?
- *Women*: Do you have children? Were the pregnancies and deliveries normal?
- Who is your medical doctor?
- When did you last have a medical check-up?

Note: For specific questions related to specific systemic problems, see Chapter 4.

Medications
- What medications do you use? How often do you take them?
- Do you use any over-the-counter medications (including aspirin)?
- Do you take any vitamins? Herbs? Other supplements?
- Do you use any type of medication patch (such as nitroglycerin, anti-smoking, or hormone patches)?
- Do you receive any type of regular injections (such as allergy shots, B-12, or hormones)?
- What pharmacy do you regularly use?

Allergies (Drugs, Inhalants, Contactants)
- Are you allergic to any medications that you know of?
- How did the medication affect you?
- Are you allergic to any eye drops we might use?
- Are you allergic to any inhalants such as pollen or dust? How do they affect you?
- Do you experience seasonal allergies?
- Do you have any allergies to foods? How does it (do they) affect you?
- Have you experienced any allergies through contact (such as lotions, rubbing alcohol, tapes, makeup? How does it (do they) affect you?

Review of Systems (ROS)

Symptom-Related Questions

Some of the symptoms may appear to be in the wrong place, such as "frequent urination," which is listed under the endocrine system. There is a reason, however. In this case, frequent urination is often a symptom of diabetes—an endocrine disorder. If you have any questions about the logic of certain questions, consult your physician/employer or a general medical text. In addition, you should add other questions, as your employer deems necessary.

Constitutional
Do you have or have you had
- unexplained weight loss or gain?
- loss or increase in appetite?
- general feeling of being unwell?
- unexplained fever?

Ears, Nose, Mouth, Throat
Do you have or have you had
- ringing in the ears?
- hearing problems?
- difficulty swallowing?
- dizziness or loss of balance?

Respiratory
Do you have or have you had
- difficulty breathing?
- shortness of breath?
- shortness of breath when walking?
- shortness of breath when lying down?
- awakened from sleep gasping for breath?
- persistent cough?
- an exposure to tuberculosis?

Endocrine

Do you have or have you had

- frequent urination?
- dry mouth?
- dizziness between meals?
- blurred vision that comes and goes?

Cardiovascular

Do you have or have you had

- irregular heart beat?
- shortness of breath?
- pain, pressure, or tightness in the chest?
- heartburn?
- dizziness?
- cold hands or feet?
- blueness in the hands or feet?

Gastrointestinal

Do you have or have you had

- a change in your bowel habits?
- black, sticky stools?
- bloody stools?
- unexplained nausea and/or vomiting?
- frequent abdominal pain?
- heartburn?

Genitourinary

Do you have or have you had

- frequent or painful urination?

Musculoskeletal

Do you have or have you had

- aching joints?
- muscle weakness?
- broken bones?
- a bad back?

Integumentary (skin)

Do you have or have you had

- any change in a mole?
- new growths?
- rashes?

Hematologic/lymphatic

Do you have or have you had

- bleeding that was difficult to stop?

- chronic lack of energy?
- swollen lymph nodes?
- blood clots?
  ### Neurological
Do you have or have you had
- tremors?
- numbness?
- weakness?
- headaches?
- seizures?
  ### Psychiatric
Do you have or have you had
- periods of the "blues" that last for more than a week or so?
- changes in your sleeping habits?
- feelings that your life is hopeless?
- thoughts of suicide?
  ### Allergic/Immunologic
Do you have or have you had
- recurrent infections?
- seasonal allergies?
- chronic runny nose and watery eyes?

System-Related Questions

  Have you had serious problems with
- your health in general?
- your ears, nose, mouth, or throat (sinus trouble)?
- your skin (skin cancer, shingles)?
- your heart (heart attack, blood pressure)?
- your blood (free bleeder, anemic)?
- your lungs (asthma, emphysema)?
- your stomach (ulcers)?
- your intestines?
- your kidneys or bladder?
- your muscles?
- your bones (arthritis)?
- your nerves (epilepsy, stroke)?
- your glands (thyroid, diabetes)?
- your immune system (leukemia, AIDS)?
- any psychiatric disorder (depression, drug dependency)?

Common Diseases and the ROS

Following is an alphabetized list of common disorders followed by the system they would fall under. Some of them could be listed under other systems; consult your practitioner as to how he or she wants such disorders labeled.

AIDS/HIV—allergic/immunologic
Albinism—constitutional
Alcoholism—psychiatric
Alzheimer's—neurologic
Anemia—hematologic/lymph
Angina—cardiovascular
Ankylosing spondylitis—musculoskeletal
Anxiety—psychiatric
Arteriosclerosis—cardiovascular
Arthritis—musculoskeletal
Asthma—respiratory
Cancer—constitutional or system involved
Carotid artery disease—cardiovascular
Chemical dependency—psychiatric
Chronic bronchitis—respiratory
Chronic obstructive pulmonary disease—respiratory
Depression—psychiatric
Diabetes—endocrine
Diverticulitis—gastrointestinal
Down syndrome—constitutional
Elevated cholesterol—constitutional or metabolic
Emphysema—respiratory
Endocarditis—cardiovascular
Epilepsy—neurologic
Goiter—endocrine
Gout—musculoskeletal
Graves' disease—endocrine
Hard of hearing—ear/nose/throat (ENT)
Hay fever—allergic/immunologic
Heart attack—cardiovascular
Heart murmur—cardiovascular
Hemophilia (free-bleeder)—hematologic/lymph
Hemorrhoids—gastrointestinal
Hepatitis—gastrointestinal (liver)
Hypertension—cardiovascular
Insomnia—constitutional
Irregular heartbeat—cardiovascular
Lupus—allergic/immunologic
Lyme disease—musculoskeletal

Migraine headaches—neurologic
Mitral valve prolapse—cardiovascular
Multiple sclerosis—musculoskeletal
Muscular dystrophy—musculoskeletal
Myasthenia gravis—endocrine
Neurofibromatosis—neurologic
Osteoporosis—musculoskeletal
Parathyroid (over- or under-active)—endocrine
Parkinson's disease—neurologic
Phlebitis—cardiovascular
Pneumonia—respiratory
Prostate cancer—genitourinary
Psoriasis—integumentary
Rheumatic fever—constitutional
Rheumatoid arthritis—musculoskeletal
Sarcoidosis—allergic/immunological
Shingles—integumentary
Sickle cell anemia—hematologic/lymph
Sickle cell disease—hematologic
Sinus problems—ENT
Stroke—neurologic
Temporal arteritis—cardiovascular
Thyroid condition—endocrine
Tinnitus (ringing in ears)—ENT
Tuberculosis—respiratory
Ulcer (stomach)—gastrointestinal
Varicose veins—cardiovascular
Vertigo—ENT

Family History

- Are there any serious illnesses or conditions that run in your family?
- Has anyone in your family had diabetes?
- Has anyone in your family had high blood pressure?
- Has anyone in your family had glaucoma?
- Has anyone in your family had cataracts?
- Has anyone in your family had macular degeneration (that's a problem in the back, inside of the eye)?
- Has anyone in your family had crossed eyes?
- Has anyone in your family had amblyopia, or "lazy eye"?
- Has anyone in your family had a retinal detachment or other retinal problems?

Social History
- Do you use tobacco products? Are you a former user?
- Do you use alcohol? Are you a former user?
- Do you use recreational drugs? Are you a former user?
- Do you live with someone?
- Tell me about your job. (What are your visual needs on the job? What are the distances to work surfaces? Do you wear eye protection?)
- What kind of hobbies do you have? (What are your visual needs for these hobbies? What are the distances to work surfaces? Do you wear eye protection?)

Special Exams

In this section, we will highlight several special types of exams that warrant different types of history questions. You will notice that, in a few cases, questions from the basic history (above) are included. This is because, while always important, these questions have special significance in the exams being discussed.

Strabismus

The New Child Patient
Ask the parent/caregiver:
- Have you noticed that an eye drifts? (If yes, When did you first notice this? Is it turned in or out? Does one eye seem to turn, or can it be either eye? Is it turned constantly, or just some of the time? If intermittent, When do you notice it? Does anything seem to make it worse? Do other people notice this as well? Do you have any photos of the child with you?)
- Do you think that he or she sees well? Does he or she seem to have any problems seeing at school? When playing sports? At home?
- Who is your pediatrician? What does he or she say about the child's eyes?
- Has anyone in the family had a crossed eye? Who? On the mother's or father's side?
- Has anyone in the family had amblyopia or "lazy eye"?

The Adult Patient
In addition to the above questions, ask the following:
- Have you had any surgery on your eye muscles in the past?
- Do you see as well out of one eye as the other?
- Did you ever wear an eye patch as a child?
- Have you ever worn glasses? (If yes, were they to help hold your eyes straight?)
    Note: See also the section on nerve palsies in Chapter 8.

Contact Lenses

The Potential Contact Lens Patient

- Have you ever tried contact lenses before? Tell me about that.
- Why do you want contact lenses?
- Do you have any specific ideas of what type of lenses you'd like?
- What type of work do you do? (What are your visual needs at work? Is this a dusty environment?)
- What type of sports and hobbies are you involved in? What are your visual needs for these activities?
- Have you ever had injury or surgery to either eye?
- Have you ever been told that you have dry eyes?
- Do you have arthritis? Thyroid problems? Hand tremors? Diabetes?
- *Women*: Do you take birth control pills? Are you pregnant or nursing?

Follow-up Exams

- How are you doing with your lenses?
- Are the lenses comfortable? Do your eyes ever feel dry? Sticky?
- Have you experienced any pain?
- Do you often feel as if there is something in your eye?
- Is your vision good? Does it change throughout the day, or is it stable? Does it change when you blink?
- Have your eyes been red?
- How many hours a day are you wearing them?
- Tell me how you're cleaning the lenses. (If disposable, how often do you put on a new pair?)

In addition, ask the new wearer:

- Are you having any problems getting your lenses in or out?
- Are you able to tell whether or not the lens is inside-out?
- Do you have any questions about the care or handling of your lenses?

Glaucoma

These questions are for the new patient who states that he or she has been previously diagnosed with glaucoma:

- How long have you known that you have glaucoma?
- Who told you that you have glaucoma?
- Did that doctor ever say what he or she thought triggered the glaucoma?
- Does anyone else in your family have glaucoma?
- Have you ever had surgery or laser for glaucoma?
- What medication(s) have you used in the past for glaucoma?

- What medication(s) are you using now? How often do you take it? When did you last use it?
- When did you last have your pressure checked? What was the reading? What does the pressure usually run?
- Have you ever had a test to check your side vision? When was the test done last? Do you have a copy?
- When did you last have a dilated exam?
- Do you have high blood pressure, anemia, or diabetes?
- Do you take medication for high blood pressure? Do you take steroids?

Elevated Intraocular Pressure (IOP)

In this scenario, a patient presents stating that his or her pressure was measured elsewhere (perhaps at a health fair screening) and was told that the IOP was elevated. Glaucoma has not actually been diagnosed in this case.
- Is there any history of glaucoma in the family?
- What type of instrument was used to measure the pressure? Was it an air-puff? Or a gadget like a big pencil? Or was a blue light used?
- Were you told the actual pressure measurement?
- Do you recall what time of day you had the test?
- When was your last regular eye exam? Do you know what the pressure was then? Do you remember whether or not your pupils were dilated?
- Have you noticed anything unusual about your eyes?
- Have you noticed anything unusual about your vision?
- As far as you can tell, has there been a decrease in your side vision?
- Do you have high blood pressure, anemia, or diabetes?
- Do you take medication for high blood pressure? Do you take steroids?

Low Vision

These are general questions about low vision suitable for the general eye care practice. For a thorough discussion on such interviewing in the low vision clinic, please see *The Low Vision Handbook* by Barbara Brown (SLACK Incorporated, 1997).
- Tell me about your eyes.
- Tell me about your vision. How long have you had low vision?
- Do you use (or have you tried) any type of visual aid (magnifiers, telescopes)? Are they satisfactory?
- Does strong lighting seem to help?
- Do you have problems with glare or light changes?
- Do you use large print? Any other type of aids?
- What things have you had to give up doing because of your vision? Which of these is the most important to you?

- Are you able to drive? If not, how do you get places?
- Are you able to keep house? Cook? Shop? Handle your business? Read your mail?
- In your daily life, what do you struggle with most because of your vision?
- What is your biggest visual challenge on the job?
- What size print do you usually encounter on the job?
- What type of hobbies do you enjoy? What type of visual challenges do these present?
- Have you been in contact with any social service agency or other group that offers help to those with low vision?
- Who helps you when you need assistance?

Patient Categories

In this section, material in parentheses indicates the nature of the problem to which that particular grouping of questions refers.

Pregnant

- How far along are you? When is the baby due?
- Do you wear contact lenses? What kind? Have you experienced any problems with them? (corneal changes due to hormones)
- Has your vision changed? (corneal changes due to hormones, retinal changes due to toxemia)
- Have you noticed any blind spots in your vision? (toxemia)
- Have you noticed that either eyelid seems drooped? (cause unknown)
- Have you noticed any change in your side vision? (pituitary hypertrophy)
- Are you diabetic?
  Note: Diabetic retinopathy can be exacerbated by pregnancy. See questions to ask a diabetic in Chapter 4.
- Have you developed toxemia? Eclampsia?
If yes:
- Have you had an increase in floaters? Noticed a curtain in your vision? (retinal detachment, vitreous heme)
- Have you experienced sudden blurred vision? Vision blackouts that come and go (lasts less than 1 minute) with normal vision between attacks? Double vision? Loss of side vision? Headache (worse in morning, worse when straining)? (papilledema)
- Have you experienced a sudden (1 to 2 days) or gradual (3 to 12 weeks) loss of vision? Blurred vision or a gray cloud that lasts 2 to 3 minutes or sometimes 30 minutes? A loss of peripheral vision? An unreactive pupil? (ischemic optic neuropathy)

Lactating

- Do you wear contact lenses? What kind? Have you experienced any problems with them? (corneal changes due to hormones)
- Has your vision changed? (corneal changes due to hormones)
- How much longer do you plan to nurse your baby?

The Premature Infant

- Tell me about the pregnancy.
- Tell me about the delivery. Was it a Cesarean section?
- How early was the baby?
- What was his or her birth weight?
- Did he or she receive oxygen? For how long?
- Did the baby have a dilated eye exam in the hospital? If so, what were the results?
- Is he or she gaining weight well? How much does the baby weigh now?
- Is the baby's growth and development normal for a premature child of this age?
- Who is your pediatrician?
- Does the baby seem to see objects?
- Does he or she follow objects with his or her eyes?
- Does he or she seem to see bright lights?
- Is there a history of any eye problems on either side of the family?

Pediatric

- Is there a history of any eye problems on either side of the family?
- Tell me about the pregnancy and delivery. Was he or she born at term?
- How much did he or she weigh at birth?
- Has his or her growth and development been normal? For example, did he or she sit at the average time, cut teeth at the average time, etc.?
- When the family is traveling in the car, does he or she seem to see distant objects at about the same time as others in the car?
- Has he or she been complaining about his or her vision or eyes?
- Does his or her eyes seem to water a lot?
- Do his or her eyes seem to move together?
- Does one eye seem to wander? In or out? All the time, or mainly when he or she is tired or sick?
- How is he or she doing in school?
- Does he or she have trouble seeing the board at school?
- Does he or she have trouble seeing to read?

- Where does he or she sit in the classroom?
- How is his or her physical coordination?
- Does he or she play sports? Have hobbies?

Menopausal

- Are you taking hormone replacement therapy?
- Have you experienced excessive tearing? Light sensitivity? Pain? Sandy/gritty sensation? Itching? Burning? Redness? (dry eye)
- Have you experienced a loss of side vision due to drooping eyelids or excess skin of the upper lids? (loss of skin and muscle tone)
- Have you experienced any foreign-body sensation and tearing? (entropion)
- Have you experienced any sagging of the lower lid? (ectropion)
- Have you experienced any headaches? (sudden development of migraine headaches, see headache section in Chapter 5)

Geriatric

- Have you experienced excessive tearing? Light sensitivity? Pain? Sandy/gritty sensation? Itching? Burning? Redness? (dry eye)
- Have you experienced a loss of side vision due to drooping eyelids or excess skin of the upper lids? (loss of skin and muscle tone)
- Have you experienced any foreign-body sensation and tearing? (entropion)
- Have you experienced any sagging of the lower lid? (ectropion)
- Have you noticed any changes in moles or other growths?
- Have you noticed the appearance of any new growths?
- Have you experienced any gradually decreased vision? Change in your color vision? Change in depth perception? Halos around lights at night? Glare from lights? Double vision? Light sensitivity? (cataracts)
- Have you noticed any loss of your central vision? (macular degeneration)
- Have you noticed any floaters? Flashes of light? (vitreous detachment)

Notes on Ocular and Systemic Medications

The *Physicians' Desk Reference*

The *Physicians' Desk Reference* (PDR) is the "bible" for information about prescription drugs. It is published every year by the Medical Economics Company and is often provided free of charge to practitioners. It can also be ordered from your neighborhood bookstore. There are other related PDR guides that are significant for those in eye care, notably *PDR Guide to Drug Interactions, Side Effects, Indications, Contraindications*; *PDR for Nonprescription Drugs*; and *PDR for Ophthalmology*. While this discussion will be focused on the PDR itself, the other guides generally follow the same format. (There are other good drug reference books available, such as the *Complete Drug Reference* by Consumer Reports and *Complete Guide to Prescription and Non-Prescription Drugs* put out by the Berkley Publishing Group. Any such book will include a section on how to look up drugs.)

The PDR is put together with the cooperation of pharmaceutical companies. It gathers, in one volume, the information found on the inserts of the various drugs. (If a company chooses not to provide this information, then the drug is not listed in the PDR.) By looking up a medication in the PDR, you can learn its correct spelling, generic name, uses, dosage, and adverse reactions. There's much more information than that, but the items I mentioned are likely to be the most useful to you during history taking.

The PDR provides several ways to find the information you want. Section 1 is the manufacturers' index. This section lists (alphabetically) all the companies whose products are listed in the book. Thus, if you remembered that Bleph-10 (Allergan, Inc., Irvine, CA)is made by Allergan, you could look up the company name and find the drug listed that way. Beside each drug is the page number on which the drug's description appears.

Section 2 (pink pages) is the brand and generic name index. Here, the drugs are listed alphabetically by both generic and trade name. So you could look up Timoptic (Merck and Co., Inc., West Point, PA) or timolol. In my experience, this is the most useful section when trying to learn about a drug during the patient history.

Section 3 (blue pages) is the product category index. This is an alphabetical listing of drugs according to what they are used for. Thus, if the patient tells you, "I'm taking a fertility drug, but I can't remember the name. I think it starts with a C," you could look up fertility agents in the blue pages. The only drug listed there that starts with a C is Clomid (Hoechst-Roussel Pharmaceuticals, Kansas City, MO), so you ask the patient if this name rings a bell. (It would be more reliable, however, to call the patient's physician or pharmacist to get the drug names whenever the patient is uncertain.)

Section 4 is the product identification guide. Included are color photos of various drugs, arranged alphabetically according to company. Some caregivers also use this section to aid in identifying what the patient is taking ("It's a pinkish-orange pill shaped like home plate"), but again it would be better to contact the patient's doctor to get the story straight.

Section 5 begins the 2,000-plus pages of product information. The drugs are arranged alphabetically according to company. The drugs of each company are then listed alphabetically under the company name. Regardless of this arrangement, it would be pretty difficult to locate any particular drug without finding it first in Section 2. Section 5 gives you all the details about the drug that we discussed above, plus a whole lot more.

Systemic Medications

Because the eye has a good blood supply, it can be particularly vulnerable to systemic medications. While there is the potential for any systemic medication to ultimately have some sort of side effect involving the eye or vision, most drugs don't cause any appreciable ocular problems. There are several, however, that are noteworthy in that they *do* tend to be associated with ocular side effects more frequently than other medications.

General Groups of Drugs

Corticosteroids
Steroids are anti-inflammatory medications. Over a period of time, systemic steroids can cause elevated intraocular pressure (IOP) in sensitive indi-

viduals. Because high IOP is not something that the patient can sense, you will not elicit this complaint on a history. However, if high IOP is sustained for a long enough period, optic atrophy, with its ocular symptoms (loss of visual acuity and color vision), can result.

Steroids can also cause posterior subcapsular cataracts. (See the cataract section in Chapter 8). Finally, steroid use has also been linked to optic neuritis and papilledema (see Chapter 8).

Chemotherapy

Chemotherapy uses various drugs to fight cancer. While the chemo attacks the cancer cells, it unfortunately also attacks healthy cells. Ocular side effects of chemo can include conjunctivitis, ocular inflammation, edema, and dry eye. Apparently, dry eye is so common in these patients that one reference suggests that all chemo patients be placed on ocular lubricants as a matter of course. (See the dry eye section in Chapter 8).

Contraceptives

Contraceptives are usually used as a method of birth control, but are also sometimes given as hormone regulators. They generally have ocular side effects similar to those of pregnancy. These include corneal changes (which may affect the fit of contact lenses) and "blind spots" in the vision (associated with migraine headaches). There is also an increased risk of retinal vessel occlusion, optic neuritis (see Chapter 8), ischemic optic neuropathy (see Chapter 8), retinal edema, and papilledema (see Chapter 8).

Antihistamines

Along with drying up sinus drainage and secretions, these medications also tend to dry out the entire body, including the eye. (See the dry eye section in Chapter 8.) Also, because of their anticholinergic action, they may also be associated with pupil dilation and blurred vision. (See the section on blurry vision in Chapter 5.) If significant pupil dilation occurs in a patient with narrow angles, an acute angle-closure glaucoma attack may occur.

Antidepressants

Antidepressants can have an anticholinergic action with associated blurry vision (see Chapter 5) and pupil dilation.

Antibiotics

Antibiotics are used to fight bacterial infections. There are many kinds, each having its own particular set of possible ocular side effects. These may include keratopathy, conjunctival inflammation, ptosis (see Chapter 8), optic neuritis (see Chapter 8), and papilledema (see Chapter 8).

Anticoagulants

These medications are given to thin the blood. As you might guess, they, therefore, have the potential to increase the risk of bleeding. Thus, patients on anticoagulants may have an increased risk of subconjunctival hemorrhage and vitreoretinal hemorrhage. A slow clotting time also has important implications in planning ocular surgery.

Salicylates (aspirin)

Aspirin is a known blood thinner and is now frequently prescribed for this reason. However, other medications that the patient may be taking might also have aspirin in them. This underscores the importance of noting *every* drug or medication that the patient may be taking, even over-the-counter ones. Table 3-1 at the end of the chapter is a list of medications that contain aspirin. In addition to their blood-thinning properties, salicylates may be associated with a disruption in the function of the extraocular muscles, so ask the patient about diplopia.

Specific Drugs

There are a few specific drugs with ocular side effects that are worth mentioning.

Plaquenil (Sanofi Winthrop, New York, NY) (hydroxychloroquine) is used in the treatment of collagen vascular diseases. Lupus and arthritis are two examples. While Plaquenil can cause deposits to form in the cornea, these deposits don't generally affect the patient's vision. However, if the deposits form in the retinal pigment epithelium, they can cause a decrease in night vision as well as a loss of central acuity. (See the poor night vision and loss of central vision sections in Chapter 5 for appropriate questions.)

Other medications that may cause ocular side effects are shown in Table 3-2 at the end of this chapter.

Topical Ocular Medications

Any medication instilled into the eye can obviously have a local effect on the eye. However, because the drug can enter the blood stream (via conjunctival capillaries), it also has access to the entire body. The drug drains through the lacrimal system as well, contacting the nasal mucosa, throat, and stomach. These all create the potential for systemic side effects.

When a patient is placed on a new ocular medication, the physician should explain any risk-producing, potential ocular and systemic side effects before the patient actually begins using it. As the history taker, your job is to be aware of the major side effects and to ask the patient about them, especially on the first visit after a new medication has been started.

You should be aware of the signs of an allergic reaction. An acute drug reaction usually occurs within 20 to 30 minutes after the drug is administered. Signs and symptoms include itching, rash, breathing problems, and a rapid, weak pulse. A local, delayed allergic reaction may occur in the eye and may include dermatitis, itching, tearing, erythema, and conjunctival edema.

Table 3-3 lists topical ocular drugs and some of their potential side effects. This information was taken from the book *Ophthalmic Medications and Pharmacology* by Duvall and Kershner, published by SLACK, Inc. When doing a history on a patient who is taking a particular type of medication, you might ask about these side effects. You can also look up the individual drugs in the *PDR Guide to Drug Interactions, Side Effects, Indications, Contraindications* and the *PDR for Ophthalmology*.

Table 3-1
Medications Containing Aspirin*

*Some of the material in this section is taken from a list in **The Crystal Clear Guide to Sight for Life** Published by Starburst Publishers, and is reprinted with permission.*

Most of the medicines listed here are named by their registered trademarks. Some are over-the-counter and some are prescription drugs. While as complete as possible, there are other aspirin-containing medications not on this list.

8-Hour Bayer Timed Release
Acuprin 81
Alka-Seltzer Original and Extra Strength
Alka-Seltzer Plus Cold Medicine
Amigesic
Anacin capsules and tablets
Anacin Maximum Strength capsules and tablets
Anaflex
Arthrinol
Arthrisin
Arthritis Pain Ascriptin
Arthritis Pain Formula (by the makers of Anacin tablets)
Arthritis Strength BC Powder
Arthritis Strength Bufferin
Arthropan
Artria SR
ASA
Ascriptin
Aspergum
Aspir-Low
Aspirin Regimen Bayer
Aspirin suppositories
Aspirtab
Astrin
Azdone
Backache Caplets
Bayer Children's Aspirin
Bayer Timed-released Aspirin
Bayer Aspirin
BC powders
Buffaprin
Bufferin
Buffex
Buffinol
Cama Arthritis Reliever
CMT
Cope
Coricidin D decongestant tablets
Coryphen
Darvon Compound-65
Disalcid
Doan's Regular Strength Tablets
Dristan decongestant
Easprin
Ecotrin tablets
Empirin, Empirin with codeine
Endodan
Entrophen
Equagesic
Excedrin
Fiorinal, Fiorinal with codeine

Gelprin
Gensan
Goody's Extra Strength Headache Powders
Halfprin
Headstart
Healthprin
Lortab
Magan
Magnaprin
Maprin
Marthritic
Measurin
Mobidin
Mono Gesic
Nervine
Night-Time Effervescent Cold
Norgesic, Norgesic Forte
Norwich Aspirin
Novasen
P-A-C Revised Formula
Panasal
Percodan, Percodan Demi tablets
Propoxyphene
Rhinocaps
Riphen
Robaxisal tablets
Roxiprin
Sal-Infant
Salatin
Saleto
Salflex
Salocol
Salsitab
Sine-Off Sinus Medicine tablets (aspirin formula)
Sloprin
Soma Compound
St. Joseph Adult Chewable
Supasa
Synalgos-DC capsules
Talwin
Therapy Bayer
Triaphen
Tricosal
Trilisate
Ursinus Inlay
Vanquish
Viro-Med tablets
YSP Aspirin Capsules
Zorprin

Table 3-2
Drugs Affecting the Eyes*

*The material in this section is taken from a list that appeared in **The Crystal Clear Guide to Sight for Life** published by Starburst Publishers, and is reprinted with permission.*

The *PDR Guide to Drug Interactions, Side Effects, Indications and Contraindications* includes listings of drugs with side effects involving the eye. These medications include oral medications, eye medications, and injected medications. Below is a list of some drugs which were found to have a certain side effect 3% or more of the time. This list is arranged alphabetically according to trade name (which are registered trademarks).

A/T/S gel- eye irritation (17 out of 90)
Accutane capsules- conjunctivitis (2 in 5), corneal opacities (5 in 72)
Anestacon solution- blurred vision, double vision
Artane- blurred vision (30-50%)
Asendin tablets- blurred vision (7%)
Bentyl- blurred vision (27%)
Buprenex injectable- small pupil (1-5%)
Cesamet pulvules- visual disturbances (13%)
Cordarone tablets- light sensitivity (4-9%), visual disturbances (4-9%)
Dilantin- jerking motions of eyes
Disopyramide phosphate CR capsules- blurred vision (3-9%), dry eye (3-9%)
Enkaid capsules- blurred vision (3.4%), visual disturbances (3.4%)
Intron A- visual disturbances (up to 7%)
Limbitrol- blurred vision
Ludiomil tablets- blurred vision (4%)
Marplan tablets- blurred vision
Mexitil capsules- blurred vision (5.7-7.5%), visual disturbances (5.7-7.5%)
Naprosyn- visual disturbances (less than 7%)
Norpace- blurred vision (3-9%), dry eyes (3-9%)
Novantrone- conjunctivitis (0-5%), eye disorders (2-7%)
Orthoclone tablets- light sensitivity (4-9%)
Permax- visual disturbances (5.8%)
Plaquenil- loss of central acuity, decrease in night vision
Quarzan capsules- blurred vision
Ridaura capsules- conjunctivitis (3-9%)
Roferon-A injection- visual disturbances (5%)
Tambocor tablets- blurred vision (15.9%), visual disturbances (15.9%)
Tegison capsules- corneal changes (10-25%), double vision, dry eye (1-10%), eye disorders (50-75%), retinal disorder (10-25%), tearing (1-10%), visual disturbances (10-25%)
Tonocard tablets- blurred vision (1.3-10%), visual disturbances (1.3-10%)
Wellbutrin tablets- blurred vision (14.6%)
Xanax tablets- blurred vision (6.2%)

Table 3-3
Ocular and Systemic Effects of Topical Ocular Drugs

DRUG TYPE	OCULAR	SYSTEMIC
Decongestant	increased redness dryness pupil dilation transient stinging	nervousness decreased heart rate headache, nervousness
Corticosteroids	PSC cataract elevated IOP (no symptoms)	stomach ulcers psychoses muscle weakness bone weakness
NSAIDS	transient stinging follicular conjunctivitis	stomach upset stomach ulcers vomiting promote asthma
Antibiotics	transient stinging allergic reaction redness photophobia depigmentation of eyelids	dermatitis digestive upset
Antivirals	transient stinging corneal toxicity	contact dermatitis
Direct-acting adrenergics	transient stinging redness	arousal of sympathetic system
Beta blockers	transient stinging	decreased heart rate slowed breathing depression confusion dizziness digestive upset headache rash insomnia impotence decreased appetite
Miotics	transient stinging blurred vision miosis accommodative spasm posterior synechiae	brow/headache sweating salivation digestive upset decreased heart rate flushing tremors difficulty breathing lethargy
Carbonic anhydrase inhibitors	conjunctival irritation	bitter taste

Systemic Disease-Related Questions

Systemic Disease

Following most questions is material in parentheses. The parenthetical notes are to indicate the possible cause of that group of symptoms in an affected individual. This is included to help you understand why a particular question (or set of questions) is important. In addition, certain questions may be repeated because they are part of a cluster of symptoms found in a certain ocular disorder. Obviously, there is no need to ask the patient the same question twice; the material is repeated so that you can learn the symptom clusters.

AIDS

- Do you seem to keep a constant eye infection? (lowered immunities)
- Have you experienced excessive tearing? Light sensitivity? Pain? Sandy/gritty sensation? Itching? Burning? Redness? (dry eye)
- Have you noticed any flat patches or raised nodules on the inside or outside of the lids? (Kaposi's sarcoma of eyelid)
- Have you noticed any flat patches or raised nodules on your eye? (Kaposi's sarcoma of conjunctiva)
- Have you experienced any light flashes? Floaters? Blurred vision? Loss of

side vision? Loss of central vision? (retinitis, spread of pneumonial infection to the choroid)
- Does your vision seem to be holding up alright, or have you noticed a slow decrease? (decreased blood flow to retina)
- Have you experienced a sudden vision loss? Vision loss that comes and goes? Decreased depth perception? Change in color vision? Pain? Loss of central vision? (optic neuritis)
- Have you experienced any double vision? (nerve palsies, involvement of bony orbit)
- Have you noticed that one or both eyes seem to protrude? (involvement of bony orbit)

Albinism

- Do you have difficulty with your vision? If you have glasses, do they help? (foveal hypoplasia, astigmatism, myopia, nystagmus)
- Has your vision changed, or does it seem fairly stable?
- Do you have problems with light sensitivity? Rate your light sensitivity on a scale of 1 to 10. (photophobia due to pigmentary dilution)
- Have you noticed any new growths on your face or any change in old growths? (increased incidence of skin malignancies)
- Do either of your eyes seem to cross? (strabismus is common)

Alcoholism

- Have you experienced double vision? Blurred vision? Droopy lid? A pupil that doesn't seem to work? (nerve palsies)
- Have you experienced a sudden vision loss? Vision loss that comes and goes? Decreased depth perception? Change in color vision? Pain? Loss of central vision? (optic neuritis)
- Have you noticed a gradual loss of vision in one eye? (alcohol amblyopia)
- Have you experienced blind spots or a blacked-out area of vision? (scotomata)

Allergies/Sinus Problems/Hay Fever

- Have you experienced redness? Excessive tearing? Glare? Light sensitivity? Headache? Matter/discharge? (ocular allergic reaction)
- Have you experienced excessive tearing? Light sensitivity? Pain? Sandy/gritty sensation? Itching? Burning? Redness? (dry eye)
- Have you had redness? Pain? Light sensitivity? Decreased vision? (iritis)

Anemia

- Have you noticed any bright red spots on the white of the eye? (subconjunctival hemorrhage)
- Have you experienced any spots or floaters? Blacked-out areas of vision? A fog or veil over your vision? A sudden loss of vision? (retinal/vitreal hemorrhage)
- Is your vision holding up, or has there been a gradual decrease? (decreased blood flow to the retina)

Ankylosing Spondylitis

- Have you had redness? Pain? Light sensitivity? Decreased vision? (acute iridocyclitis)
- Have you had decreased or distorted vision? (macular edema)
- Does your vision seem to get worse in situations where there is glare? (posterior subcapsular cataract due to repeated inflammation)

Arteriosclerosis

- Have you experienced any spots or floaters? Blacked-out areas of vision? A fog or veil over your vision? A sudden loss of vision? (retinal/vitreal hemorrhage)
- Have you experienced any decreased vision? (retinal edema)
- Have you noticed a loss of central reading vision? (macular degeneration)

Asthma

- Have you experienced any redness? Excessive tearing? Light sensitivity? (conjunctivitis)
- Have you experienced any gradually decreased vision? Change in your color vision? Change in depth perception? Halos around lights at night? Glare from lights? Double vision? Light sensitivity? (cataracts secondary to steroid treatment)

Cancer

- Have you experienced any blurred vision? Loss of vision? Loss of peripheral vision? Double vision? (spread of cancer to eye)
- Have you noticed any new growths? Protrusion of the eye? (spread of cancer to eye)
- Have you had any eye pain? Redness? (spread of cancer to eye)

Carotid Artery Disease

- Have you had redness? Pain? Light sensitivity? Decreased vision? (iritis)
- Have your eyes been red, without other symptoms of pain or discharge? (swelling of conjunctival blood vessels)
- Have you experienced any spots or floaters? Blacked-out areas of vision? A fog or veil over your vision? A sudden loss of vision? (retinal/vitreal hemorrhage)
- Is your vision holding up, or has there been a gradual decrease? (decreased blood flow to the retina)

Chicken Pox

- Have any lesions appeared on the lids? Where (on the skin of the lid or on the lid margin)?
- Is the eye red and inflamed?
- Does the patient seem to have or complain of eye pain? (keratitis)

Diabetes

- How long have you been a diabetic?
- How do you control your sugar level?
- When did you last take your medication?
- When did you last have your sugar level checked? What was the reading?
- Does your sugar level seem to be stable, or does it fluctuate?
- Do you have episodes of blurred vision that come and go? (blood sugar fluctuations)
- Have you had any double vision? (nerve palsies)
- Have you experienced any gradually decreased vision? Change in your color vision? Change in depth perception? Halos around lights at night? Glare from lights? Double vision? Light sensitivity? (cataracts)
- Have you experienced any spots or floaters? Blacked-out areas of vision? A fog or veil over your vision? A sudden loss of vision? (retinal/vitreal hemorrhage)
- Is your vision holding up, or has there been some decrease? (exudates, decreased retinal blood flow, neovascularization)
- Have you experienced a sudden vision loss? Vision loss that comes and goes? Decreased depth perception? Change in color vision? Pain? Loss of central vision? (optic neuritis)
- Have you experienced any sudden vision losses? (optic atrophy)
- Have you experienced blurry areas of vision? Blurred vision? (retinal vein occlusion)

Down Syndrome

This interview plan assumes that you will be asking the questions of a care-giver, although that may not always be the case
- Have you noticed crusting and/or redness of the lid margins? (blepharitis)
- Is there frequent tearing? (nasolacrimal duct obstruction, infantile glaucoma)
- Is there any type of discharge that won't seem to clear up? (nasolacrimal duct obstruction)
- Does he or she seem to be light sensitive? (infantile glaucoma)
- Does he or she tend to hold objects very close in order to see them? (high myopia)
- Does he or she seem to rub the eyes a lot? (blepharitis, keratoconus)
- Does either eye seem to cross or drift? (strabismus)
- Does he or she tend to constantly tilt the head? (astigmatism)
- Does the pupil look cloudy? (retinoblastoma, cataract)
- Does the front of the eye ever look cloudy? (corneal edema)

Emphysema

- Have you experienced any gradually decreased vision? Change in your color vision? Change in depth perception? Halos around lights at night? Glare from lights? Double vision? Light sensitivity? (cataracts secondary to steroid treatment)

Endocarditis

- Have you noticed any bright red spots on the white of the eye? (subconjunctival hemorrhage)
- Have you experienced any spots or floaters? Blacked-out areas of vision? A fog or veil over your vision? A sudden loss of vision? (retinal/vitreal hemorrhage)
- Have you experienced double vision? Blurred vision? Droopy lid? A pupil that doesn't seem to work? (nerve palsies)
- Have you had redness? Pain? Light sensitivity? Decreased vision? (iritis)
- Have you experienced any generalized vision loss? A loss of peripheral vision? (papillitis)
- Is your vision holding up, or has there been some decrease? (decreased retinal blood flow)
- Have you experienced sudden pain? Redness? Lid swelling? Lid twitching? A loss of vision? (metastatic endophthalmitis)

Gonorrhea

- Have you had a discharge from your eyes? (copious mucopurulent discharge secondary to conjunctivitis)
- Have your eyes been red? (conjunctivitis)
- Have your lids been swollen? (conjunctivitis)
- Is the area right in front of your ear(s) swollen and tender? (positive pre-auricular nodes associated with conjunctivitis)
- Have you had redness? Pain? Decreased vision? (iridocyclitis, endophthalmitis)
- Do you feel as if something is in your eye or that your eyelid is rubbing every time you blink? (corneal ulcer)

Gout

- Have you experienced redness? Pain (usually when moving the eye)? Tearing? Sensitivity to light? (episcleritis)
- Have you experienced redness? A deep ache or pain? Light sensitivity? Tearing? Decreased vision? (scleritis)
- Have you experienced halos around lights? Starbursts from lights? Light sensitivity? (crystals in cornea)
- Have you experienced redness? Pain? Light sensitivity? Tearing? Blurred vision? (iritis)

Graves' Disease

- Have you noticed any change in the skin color of your eyelids? (increased pigmentation)
- Have people commented that you seem to be staring? (intermittent stare)
- Does it seem as if your upper lids are higher than they used to be? (lid retraction)
- Have you noticed that one or both eyes seem to bulge out? (exophthalmos)
- Do your lids or the area around your eyes seem to be puffy? (lid or orbital edema)
- Have you experienced any double vision? (muscle weakness or palsy)
- Have you noticed any increased tearing? (dryness)
- Do you ever feel as if your eyes have sand or grit in them? (dryness, corneal involvement)

Herpes Simplex

- Have you noticed any lesions on your eyelids? (vesicles)
- Have you noticed any crusting on your eyelids? (blepharitis)

- Have you had any redness? Discharge? (conjunctivitis)
- Have you noticed any redness? Pain? Decreased vision? (keratitis, iritis)
- Have you had the sensation as if there is something in your eye or that your eyelid rubs the eye every time you blink? (corneal ulcer, keratitis)
- Have you had any swelling of the lids and/or area around the eye(s)? (cellulitis)

Hypertension

- How long have you had high blood pressure?
- How do you control it?
- Have you experienced any spots or floaters? Blacked-out areas of vision? A fog or veil over your vision? A sudden loss of vision? (retinal/vitreal hemorrhage)
- Have you experienced any decreased vision? (retinal edema)
- Have you experienced sudden blurred vision? Vision blackouts that come and go (lasts less than 1 minute) with normal vision between attacks? Double vision? Loss of side vision? Headache (worse in morning, worse when straining)? (papilledema)
- Is your vision holding up, or has there been some decrease? (exudates)

Leukemia

- Have you noticed any protrusion of the eye(s)? (presence of periorbital leukemia cells)
- Have you experienced any spots or floaters? Blacked-out areas of vision? A fog or veil over your vision? A sudden loss of vision? (retinal/vitreal hemorrhage)
- Have you experienced any floaters? (leukemia cells in aqueous)
- Have you experienced any episodes of sudden vision loss (may occur over a period of several hours)? (leukemia cells clogging optic nerve)
- Have you experienced any decreased vision? (retinal edema, exudates)
- Have you experienced any generalized vision loss? A loss of peripheral vision? (papillitis)
- Have you experienced any sudden appearance (over a period of 1 to 2 days) of pain? Redness? Lid swelling? Lid twitching? Loss of vision? (metastatic endophthalmitis)

Lupus

- Have you experienced any spots or floaters? Blacked-out areas of vision? A fog or veil over your vision? A sudden loss of vision? (retinal/vitreal hemorrhage)

- Have you experienced any decreased vision? (retinal edema, exudates)
- Have you noticed any round marks or redness on the skin of your lids? (dermatologic changes)
- Have you experienced any pain? Scratchiness or foreign-body sensation? Light sensitivity? Decreased vision? Tearing? (keratitis)
- Have you experienced redness? Pain? Light sensitivity? Tearing? Blurred vision? (iritis)

Lyme Disease

- Have you had any sensitivity to light? (photophobia)
- Have the eyes been red? (conjunctivitis without discharge)
- Have you experienced redness? Pain? Light sensitivity? Tearing? Blurred vision? (iritis)
- Have you experienced any distorted vision? (macular edema)
- Have you experienced any lid twitching? (blepharospasm)
- Have you noticed a red spot on either eye, perhaps accompanied by pain? (episcleritis)
- Have you experienced a sudden vision loss? Vision loss that comes and goes? Decreased depth perception? Change in color vision? Pain? Loss of central vision? (optic neuritis)
- Have you experienced any sudden vision loss? (optic atrophy)

Malnutrition

- Have you noticed any lid swelling or a sensation of fullness in your eyes?
- Have you experienced excessive tearing? Light sensitivity? Pain? Sandy/gritty sensation? Itching? Burning? Redness? (dry eye)
- Have you noticed any problems with seeing in dim lighting? (night blindness)

Measles

- Have you had any redness? Was it accompanied by discomfort? Discharge? Itching? (conjunctivitis)
- Have you noticed any spots on your eye? (Koplik's spot)

Migraine Headaches

- Do you ever notice "blind spots" in your vision?
- Do you ever experience a loss or closing in of side vision?
- Do you ever see jagged lights around your vision?
- Are these visual symptoms followed by a headache?

Note: These symptoms are caused by spasms of the blood vessels. For further questions, see Headaches, Chapter 5.

Mitral Valve Prolapse

- Have you ever experienced a total loss of vision? (retinal artery occlusion due to platelet emboli)
- Have you experienced sudden, painless loss of vision in one eye, where the vision came back in 2 to 10 minutes? (amaoursis fugax caused by transient ischemic attacks)

Multiple Sclerosis

- Have you experienced a sudden vision loss? Vision loss that comes and goes? Decreased depth perception? Change in color vision? Pain? Loss of central vision? (optic neuritis)
- Have you ever noticed jerking movements of your eyes? Have you experienced blurred vision or noticed that objects seem to move or vibrate? (nystagmus)
- Have you experienced double vision? (muscle weakness, nerve palsy)
- Have you experienced drooping of the upper lid? Noticed that one pupil was larger than the other? (nerve palsy)

Muscular Dystrophy

- Have you noticed any double vision? Lid droop? (muscle deterioration)
- Have you experienced excessive tearing? Light sensitivity? Pain? Sandy/gritty sensation? Itching? Burning? Redness? (dry eye)
- Have you experienced any gradually decreased vision? Change in your color vision? Change in depth perception? Halos around lights at night? Glare from lights? Double vision? Light sensitivity? (cataracts)

Myasthenia Gravis

- Have you ever noticed jerking movements of your eyes? Have you experienced blurred vision or noticed that objects seem to move or vibrate? (nystagmus)
- Have you experienced double vision? (muscle weakness, nerve palsy)
- Have you experienced drooping of the upper lid? (nerve palsy)
- Have you noticed that one pupil was larger than the other? (nerve palsy)

Neurofibromatosis (von Recklinghausen's disease)

- Have you noticed any protrusion of the eye(s)? Drooping lids? Thickened lids? Tumors on your lids?
- Have you experienced any vision loss? A loss of your peripheral vision? These changes are all caused by the presence of neurofibromas.

Occlusive Vascular Disease (Sudden)

- Have you had episodes where your vision goes out and then comes back? (clots moving through blood vessels inside the eye)
- Have you experienced any sudden loss of vision? (blockage of retinal blood vessels)

Parathyroid (Overactive)

- Have you experienced any pain? Scratchiness or foreign-body sensation? Light sensitivity? Decreased vision? Tearing? (keratitis)
- Have you experienced any foreign-body sensation? Scratchiness? Tearing? (calcium deposits in conjunctiva)
- Have you experienced halos around lights? Starbursts from lights? Light sensitivity? (crystals in cornea)

Parathyroid (Underactive)

- Have you experienced any redness? Excessive tearing? Light sensitivity? (conjunctivitis)
- Have you experienced any pain? Scratchiness or foreign-body sensation? Light sensitivity? Decreased vision? Tearing? (keratitis)
- Have you experienced any gradually decreased vision? Change in your color vision? Change in depth perception? Halos around lights at night? Glare from lights? Double vision? Light sensitivity? (cataracts)
- Have you experienced sudden blurred vision? Vision blackouts that come and go (last less than 1 minute) with normal vision between attacks? Double vision? Loss of side vision? Headache (worse in morning, worse when straining)? (papilledema)

Pituitary Adenoma

- Have you noticed any problems with your peripheral vision? (bi-temporal field loss)
- Have you had any double vision? (EOM palsies)
- Have you noticed any protruding of one or both eyes? (proptosis)
- Have you experienced a sudden loss of vision? (pituitary hemorrhage)

Psoriasis

- Have you experienced any redness? Excessive tearing? Light sensitivity? (conjunctivitis)
- Have you experienced itching of the lids? Lid swelling? Crusting lids? (blepharitis)
- Have you experienced any pain? Scratchiness or foreign-body sensation? Light sensitivity? Decreased vision? Tearing? (keratitis)

Rheumatoid Arthritis

- Have you experienced excessive tearing? Light sensitivity? Pain? Sandy/gritty sensation? Itching? Burning? Redness? (dry eye)
- Have you experienced any redness? Excessive tearing? Light sensitivity? (conjunctivitis)
- Have you experienced redness? Pain (usually when moving the eye)? Tearing? Sensitivity to light? (episcleritis)
- Have you experienced redness? A deep ache or pain? Light sensitivity? Tearing? Decreased vision? (scleritis)
- Have you experienced redness? Pain? Light sensitivity? Tearing? Blurred vision? (iritis)
- Have you experienced any gradually decreased vision? Change in your color vision? Change in depth perception? Halos around lights at night? Glare from lights? Double vision? Light sensitivity? (cataracts secondary to steroid treatment)

Sarcoidosis

- Have you experienced redness? Pain? Light sensitivity? Tearing? Blurred vision? (iritis)
- Have you experienced any pain? Redness? Light sensitivity? Blurred vision? (uveitis)
- Have you experienced any mild pain? Mild light sensitivity? Mild blurred vision? (chorioretinitis)

Shingles

- Have you developed any pain? Lid droop? Lid swelling? Lid redness? (lesions on skin)
- Have you experienced any excessive tearing? Light sensitivity? Pain? Sandy/gritty sensation? Itching? Burning? Redness? (lid paralysis/incomplete lid closure)
- Have you experienced any double vision? (nerve palsies)

- Have you experienced redness? A deep ache or pain? Light sensitivity? Tearing? Decreased vision? (scleritis)
- Have you experienced any pain? Scratchiness or foreign-body sensation? Light sensitivity? Decreased vision? Tearing? (keratitis)
- Have you experienced any blurred vision? Halos around lights? Light sensitivity? (corneal edema)
- Have you experienced redness? Pain? Light sensitivity? Tearing? Blurred vision? (iritis)
- Have you experienced a sudden vision loss? Vision loss that comes and goes? Decreased depth perception? Change in color vision? Pain? Loss of central vision? (optic neuritis)

Sickle Cell Disease

- Have you noticed any bulging of the eye(s)? (proptosis)
- Have you had an increase in floaters? A curtain in your vision? (retinal detachment, vitreous heme)
- Have you noticed any "blind spots" in your vision? (retinal holes)
- Have you experienced sudden blurred vision? Vision blackouts that come and go (last less than 1 minute) with normal vision between attacks? Double vision? Loss of side vision? Headache (worse in morning, worse when straining)? (papilledema)

Smoking

- Have you experienced any sudden vision loss? (optic atrophy)
- Have you noticed a gradual loss of vision in one eye? (tobacco amblyopia)
- Have you experienced any gradually decreased vision? Change in your color vision? Change in depth perception? Halos around lights at night? Glare from lights? Double vision? Light sensitivity? (cataracts)
- Are you diabetic? (Smoking increases the risk of diabetic retinal disease.)
- Have you noticed any loss of your central vision? (increased incidence of macular degeneration)
- Have you experienced excessive tearing? Light sensitivity? Pain? Sandy/gritty sensation? Itching? Burning? Redness? (dry eye)

Syphilis

- Have you experienced any pain? Scratchiness or foreign-body sensation? Light sensitivity? Decreased vision? Tearing? (keratitis)
- Have you experienced redness? A deep ache or pain? Light sensitivity? Tearing? Decreased vision? (scleritis)
- Have you experienced redness? Pain? Light sensitivity? Tearing? Blurred vision? (iritis)
- Have you experienced any pain? Redness? Light sensitivity? Blurred vision? (uveitis)

- Have you experienced a sudden vision loss? A vision loss that comes and goes? Decreased depth perception? Change in color vision? Pain? Loss of central vision? (optic neuritis)
- Have you experienced sudden blurred vision? Vision blackouts that come and go (last less than 1 minute) with normal vision between attacks? Double vision? Loss of side vision? Headache (worse in morning, worse when straining)? (papilledema)

Temporal (Giant Cell) Arteritis

- Have you experienced any double vision or lid droop? (nerve palsies)
- Have you experienced redness? Pain? Light sensitivity? Tearing? Blurred vision? (iritis)
- Have you experienced any spots or floaters? Blacked-out areas of vision? A fog or veil over your vision? A sudden loss of vision? (retinal/vitreal hemorrhage)
- Have you experienced a total loss of vision? (retinal artery occlusion)
- Have you experienced a sudden vision loss? A vision loss that comes and goes? Decreased depth perception? Change in color vision? Pain? Loss of central vision? (optic neuritis)
- Have you experienced a sudden (1 to 2 days) or gradual (3 to 12 weeks) loss of vision? Vision loss that comes and goes (blurred vision or a gray cloud that lasts 2 to 3 minutes or sometimes 30 minutes)? Loss of peripheral vision? An unreactive pupil? (ischemic optic neuropathy)
- Have you experienced a gradual loss of vision? (exudates)

Thyroid (Overactive)—Graves' Disease

- Have you noticed any protrusion of the eye(s)? Puffiness around the eyes? Incomplete closure of the eyelids?
- Have you experienced excessive tearing? Light sensitivity? Pain? Sandy/gritty sensation? Itching? Burning? Redness? (dry eye from incomplete lid closure)
- Have you experienced any sudden vision loss? (optic atrophy)
- Have you experienced sudden blurred vision? Vision blackouts that come and go (last less than 1 minute) with normal vision between attacks? Double vision? Loss of side vision? Headache (worse in morning, worse when straining)? (papilledema)

Thyroid (Underactive)

- Have you noticed any swelling around your eyes? Eyelid swelling? A loss of the outer third of your eyebrows?
- Have you experienced any gradually decreased vision? Change in your color vision? Change in depth perception? Halos around lights at night? Glare from lights? Double vision? Light sensitivity? (cataracts)
- Have you experienced a sudden vision loss? A vision loss that comes and goes? Decreased depth perception? Change in color vision? Pain? Loss of central vision? (optic neuritis)
- Have you experienced any sudden vision loss? (optic atrophy)

Tuberculosis

- Have you experienced redness? A deep ache or pain? Light sensitivity? Tearing? Decreased vision? (scleritis)
- Have you experienced a sudden vision loss? Vision loss that comes and goes? Decreased depth perception? Change in color vision? Pain? Loss of central vision? (optic neuritis)
- Have you experienced any pain? Redness? Light sensitivity? Blurred vision? (uveitis)

Note: Much of the material in this chapter is taken from *The Crystal Clear Guide to Sight for Life* (Starburst Publishers), and has been reprinted with permission of the publisher.

Symptom-Related Questions

This chapter is divided into two sections. Section one (starts on this page) discusses symptoms of a visual nature. Section two lists physical symptoms. Symptoms are listed alphabetically. If you don't find a particular item, try wording it a different way (for example, "flashing lights" is listed as "light flashes").

Following each symptom is a list of questions to ask the patient. After the questions is a list of possible causes of each symptom. This list is included to help you understand what may be happening to the patient.

Section One: Visual Symptoms

Blurry Vision

- When did the blurred vision start?
- Did it begin gradually and get worse slowly, or was it sudden?
- Is it blurred only in the distance? Only close up? Or both?
- Does the blurring come and go?
- Is it in one eye or both?
- Is it a general blurring or just in a certain spot (like a cloud or a curtain)?
- Do your glasses make it better or worse? How old are your glasses?
    Possible causes: change in glasses prescription, cataract, blood sugar fluctu-

ations, diabetes, poor blood pressure control, drug reaction, angle-closure glaucoma, retinal detachment, inflammation inside the eye, fatigue, hunger, vitamin deficiency, hormonal disorders, fainting, heart failure, arteriosclerosis, large floater

Color Vision, Change in

- When did you first notice the change?
- Have both eyes changed or just one?
- Are colors brighter or more dull?
- What colors seem to be most affected? Greens? Blues and purples?
- Have you been told that you have cataracts?
- Have you recently had cataract surgery?
- Have you recently been exposed to bright lights or high glare (off of snow, sand, or water)?
- Are you taking Placquinil (hydroxychloroquine)?
- Is there a family history of color blindness?
   Possible causes: cataracts, drug reaction, diabetes, glaucoma, retina or macular disease

Curtain over the Vision

- When did you first notice the curtain?
- Which eye is affected?
- Can you see through the curtain, or is it solid?
- Where does the curtain seem to be coming from: the top, bottom?
- Have you had a blow to the eye?
- Have you had any type of eye surgery?
- Have you seen any light flashes?
- Does the curtain move around when you move your eye?
   Possible causes: retinal detachment, posterior vitreous detachment, hemorrhage

Distorted Vision

- When did you first notice this?
- Is the distortion in one eye or both?
- Is it constant, or does it come and go?
- Describe the distortion. (Parts of words missing or crooked, round objects appear oblong, straight lines appear wavy, etc.)
   Possible causes: macular degeneration, astigmatism, inflammation inside the eye, retinal detachment or hole

Double Vision (Diplopia)

- When did the double vision start? What were you doing at the time?
- Did you experience any dizziness or weakness when it started?
- Is your vision double all the time or just some of the time?
- Is your vision doubled when you look into the distance, up close, or both?
- Is the second image above, to the side, or at an angle from the first image?
- Does the double image go away if you cover one eye?
- Does the double image go away or get worse if you tilt or turn your head a certain way?
- Is your vision doubled with your glasses, without, or both?
- Could your glasses be out of line? Have you just gotten new glasses?
- Is the double vision associated with a headache?
- Have you been told that you have a cataract?
- Have you had a head injury?
- Are you diabetic?
- Do you take vitamin A? How much?

   Possible causes: Paralysis of one or more of the muscles that move the eye, misaligned glasses, cataract, dislocation of intraocular lens implant, head trauma, dislocation of the lens, fluid behind the eye, fracture of the bones around the eye, large difference in glasses correction between the eyes, stroke, multiple sclerosis, thyroid trouble, diabetes, vitamin toxicity, giant cell arteritis, myasthenia gravis

Fluctuating Vision

- How long has this been going on?
- .Does this occur in one eye or both?
- Does it occur with or without glasses, or both?
- Does the vision just get blurry, or does it black out?
- Do you have diabetes?
- When did you last have your blood sugar checked?
- Is there a history of diabetes in the family?
- Have you been told that you have cataracts?
- Have you had any type of eye surgery?
- Do you use any type of eye drops or ointment?
- Do you have any type of discharge from the eyes?
- When does the blurring occur? (Just in the mornings, or mostly when reading?)

   Possible causes: diabetic blood sugar fluctuations, cataracts, ointment or matter in the eye, dry eyes, blood vessel disease

Glare

- How long has this been bothering you?
- Does your vision worsen in bright sunlight?
- Are you having a problem with headlights from oncoming cars at night?
- Have you been told that you have cataracts?
- Have you had cataract surgery?
    Possible causes: cataract, corneal scar or dystrophy, capsule opacity after cataract surgery, drug reaction

Halos (Around Lights at Night)

- How long have you noticed this?
- Is it happening in one eye or both?
- Have you been told that you have cataracts?
- Is the eye ever painful?
- Are you having headaches?
- Is the eye ever red?
- Do you notice this all the time or just now and then?
    Possible causes: glaucoma, cataracts, mucus on the cornea, corneal scar, drug reaction, exposure to intense light, dislocated intraocular lens implant, corneal edema

Improvement of Near Vision

(Patient notices that he or she doesn't need reading glasses anymore, when he or she used to have to have them.)
- When did you first notice this?
- Has it been a gradual change?
- Is it in one eye or both?
- Have you been told that you have cataracts?
- Have you had cataract surgery?
    Possible causes: cataracts, cloudy capsule after cataract surgery

Light Flashes

- When did this start?
- How often do you see the flashes?
- How long does it last? A second? Thirty minutes?
- Is it constant, or does it come and go?
- Describe the flashes (lightning streaks, jagged, saw-toothed, sparkling, colored, etc.).
- Which eye is affected?

- Have you also had any floaters (specks)? Spots? Curtains?
- Do you see the lights even with your eyes closed?
- Have you had a blow to the eye?
- Have you had eye surgery?
- Has your vision been affected?
- Do you have a headache after the lights disappear?

    Possible causes: posterior vitreous detachment, retinal detachment or tear, migraine headache, ocular migraine (without headache), brain concussion, glaucoma

Loss of Central Vision

- When did you first notice this?
- Did your vision fade out gradually or go out suddenly?
- Does this come and go, or is it constant?
- Is your center vision totally blacked out or just foggy?
- Did you have a headache after this occurred?

    Possible causes: stroke, central retinal artery or vein occlusion, macular degeneration, retinal tear or hole, migraine, drug reaction, nutritional deficiency

Loss of Depth Perception

- When did you first notice this?
- Have you recently lost vision in one eye?
- Is your vision good in one eye and poor in the other?
- Have you been told that you have cataracts?

    Possible causes: cataract, difference in vision between the two eyes, loss of vision in one eye

Loss of Near Vision

- When did you first notice this?
- Has it changed gradually or suddenly?
- Is it in one eye or both?
- Is it with your glasses on? Off? Or both?
- Is it constant, or does it come and go?
- What exactly have you noticed that you are unable to see? The newspaper or phone book? Threading a needle? The speedometer? Something on a grocery shelf?
- Are you using any type of eye drop with a red top?

    Possible causes: age, need for glasses change, accommodative spasms (in young people), cataract, drug reaction

Loss of Side (Peripheral) Vision

- When did you first notice this?
- Is it in both eyes or just one?
- Does it come and go, or is it constant?
- Have you noticed any flashes of light?
- Have you had a blow to the eye?
- Has this been accompanied by any dizziness, headaches, weakness, etc.?
- Have you been told that you have glaucoma?
    Possible causes: retinal detachment, glaucoma, pituitary tumor, stroke

Loss of Upper Field of Vision

- When did you first notice this?
- Is it in one eye or both?
- Does it come and go, or is it constant?
- Have you noticed any flashes of light?
- Have you had a blow to the eye?
- Has this been accompanied by any dizziness, headache, weakness, etc.?
- Is extra skin from your upper lids hanging down into your eyes?
    Possible causes: drooping eyelids, retinal detachment, basilar artery insufficiency, optic neuritis

Loss of Vision (Gradual)

- When did you first notice the decrease?
- Describe in detail how your vision is decreased.
- Is the decrease in one eye or both?
- Is the decrease constant, or does it come and go?
- Do you notice this more close up (for reading) or at a distance?
- When did you last have your glasses changed?
- Do you take vitamin B? How much?
    Possible causes: need to change glasses, cataracts, diabetes, vitamin toxicity, drug reaction

Loss of Vision (Sudden)

- When did you first notice this?
- Which eye is affected?
- Is your vision totally blacked out in that eye, or can you see light? Movement?
- Do you have hardening of the arteries?
- Is the eye painful?

- Is the eye red?
- Have you had injury or surgery to the eye?
  Possible causes: angle-closure glaucoma, stroke, brain injury, retinal detachment, temporal arteritis, hemorrhage inside the eye, drug reaction, optic nerve disease, blockage of vein or artery inside eye, psychological

Poor Distant Vision (Where near vision remains good)

- How long has this been bothering you?
- Is it in one eye or both?
- Is it constant, or does it come and go?
- Do you wear glasses? Do they help?
- When was the last time you had your glasses changed?
  Possible causes: uncorrected refractive error, cataract

Poor Near Vision (Where distant vision remains good)

- How long has this been bothering you?
- Is it in one eye or both?
- Is it constant, or does it come and go?
- Do you wear glasses? Do they help?
- Does a magnifying glass help?
- When was the last time you had your glasses changed?
  Possible causes: uncorrected refractive error, presbyopia, macular degeneration

Poor Night Vision

- When did this start?
- Is there a history of night blindness in the family?
- Does anyone in the family have retinitis pigmentosa?
- Are you mainly bothered by glare from oncoming headlights at night?
  Possible causes: cataracts, retinitis pigmentosa, malnutrition (vitamin A deficiency), advanced glaucoma

Specks Before the Eyes (Floaters)

- When did you first notice the floaters?
- Is it in one eye or both?
- When do you see them?
- Describe the shape: spider-web, dust-like, hair, specks/bugs, a circle or half-moon, a curtain, a spot?
- Have you had a blow to the eye?
- Have you had eye surgery?

- Do they scoot around when you move your eye or stay in the same place?
- Has your vision decreased?
- Have the floaters increased in number or size since you first noticed them?
- Have you seen any light flashes?
    Possible causes: retinal detachment, retinal hemorrhage, posterior vitreous detachment, high nearsightedness (myopia)

Starbursts from Headlights

- When did this start?
- Is it constant, or does it come and go?
- Have you been told that you have cataracts?
- Have you had cataract surgery?
- Have you had corneal surgery?
- Do you have astigmatism?
- Have you had a corneal injury?
- Does this occur with your glasses on? Off? Or both?
    Possible causes: cataracts, uncorrected astigmatism, capsule opacity, displaced intraocular lens, corneal scar, glaucoma

Uncomfortable Vision (Asthenopia)

- When did this start?
- Is it in one eye or both?
- Is the discomfort constant, or does it come and go? Does it occur during a certain part of the day?
- Describe the discomfort. (Examples: tired feeling, drawing, "just not right")
- How long has it been since you had your glasses changed?
- Have you recently had your glasses changed?
    Possible causes: eye strain, need glasses changed, incorrect prescription, eye muscle imbalance, glasses need adjusting

Problems with New Glasses

- How long have you had the new glasses?
- How much have you been wearing them?
- Have you gone back to wearing your old glasses since getting the new?
- Did you have one lens changed or both?
- Is this your first pair of bifocals or trifocals?

Vision Problems

• Are you having trouble seeing at distance? At near? Or both?
  Distance: Is it better if you lift the glasses up or down a bit? If you tilt the frames on your face? If you tuck your chin?
  Near: Is the print any clearer if you hold the material closer or farther back? If you lift the glasses up or down? If you lift your chin while looking down?

Discomfort

• Please describe the discomfort. (Examples: tired feeling, pulling sensation, headache, "just not right")
• Are the frames uncomfortable? Where do they bother you?

Distortion

• Do you notice the distortion in one eye or both?
• Do you notice this at distance, near, or both?
• Do lines seem to bow in or out?
• Did you go from plastic lenses to glass or from glass to plastic?
  Possible causes: Regretfully, the possible causes of problems with new glasses are beyond the scope of this book. The questions listed above are based on optical principles. For a complete discussion of the topic, please consult *Exercises in Refractometry*, published by SLACK Incorporated.

Section Two: Physical Symptoms

Burning

• How long has this been bothering you?
• What time of day is it worse? If it starts early in the morning, does it get better during the day?
• Does this happen when you are doing a certain activity (such as reading or watching TV)?
• Do you tend to have seasonal or environmental allergies?
• Do your eyes also water? Itch?
• Have you tried any kind of eye drops to clear this up? Did it help?
• Are you taking any kind of antihistamines, sinus, cold, or allergy medication?
  Possible causes: dry eyes, staring (forgetting to blink while reading or watching TV), allergy, drug reaction

Crossed/Drifting Eye

• When did you first notice this?

- Which eye seems to be crossing? If both, does one seem to drift more than the other?
- Does the eye cross in, out, up, or down?
- Does the eye cross all the time? If not, when does it seem to cross more?
- Are you having any double vision? Are the images vertical, horizontal, or offset?
- Has your vision changed in either eye?
- Are there any associated symptoms, such as headache, dizziness, etc.?
- Is there a family history of crossed eyes?
- Have you had a head injury?
- Have you had eye surgery?
- Are you diabetic?
- Do you have any type of muscular disorder?
- Do you have an old photograph with you? (evaluate for presence of strabismus in photo)

Possible causes: congenital strabismus, decompensating phoria, head injury, muscle weakness, nerve palsy

Crusting Lids

- When did this start?
- Is it in one eye or both?
- Are your eyes matted shut in the morning?
- Are the crusts on your lashes? Or just in the corners of your eyes?
- Is there any redness? Watering? Itching? Burning? Pain?
- Has your vision changed?
- Have you tried treating this yourself? How? Did it help?
- Are you diabetic?
- Do you have any skin disorders (such as seborrhea, rosacea, etc.)?

Possible causes: low-grade lid infection (blepharitis), infection, diabetes, seborrhea, rosacea

Difference in Pupil Size

- When did you first notice this?
- Do you use a green-top drop in one eye?
- Do you use a red-top drop in one eye?
- Have you had an injury?
- Have you had any type of eye surgery?
- Is the vision in either eye blurred?
- Is the eye with the smaller pupil sensitive to light? Red?
- Is the eye with the larger pupil sensitive to light? Red? Is it painful? Do you

have blurred vision?
- Does the eyelid droop in the eye with the smaller pupil?

Possible causes: congenital (born with it), angle-closure glaucoma, surgery, trauma, inflammation inside the eye, drug reaction (pharmaceutical), optic nerve damage, Horner's syndrome

Growths

- When did you first notice the growth?
- Has it changed? Grown rapidly? Changed color? Have more growths come up?
- Does the growth ever bleed? Ooze or weep? Crust over?
- Have you tried to treat it yourself?
- Is the growth tender and sore?
- Have you ever had any type of skin cancer?

Possible causes: mole, allergic reaction, xanthelasma, stye, chalazion, skin cancer, wart, cyst

Headaches

- How long has this been bothering you?
- What part of your head hurts?
- How long does the headache last?
- How often do you have a headache?
- What time of day do the headaches occur?
- Are the headaches associated with reading or close work?
- Do the headaches seem to be associated with certain foods or alcohol?
- Have you taken any medication to relieve it? Did that help?
- What activities make the headache better (such as taking a nap)? Worse?
- Is the headache centered around one eye? If so, does the eye turn red and the vision decrease when it hurts?
- Does it hurt worse when you bend over?
- Do you have high blood pressure?
- Is there a rash on your forehead?
- Are you using any type of eye drops?
- Have you just started any new medication?

Possible causes: angle-closure glaucoma, migraine, sinus, eye muscle imbalance, drug reaction, shingles, high blood pressure

Itching

- When did this start?
- Is it in one eye or both?

- Does this seem to recur at the same time every year?
- Do you tend to have allergies?
- Where does it itch? (Example: lids, edge of lids, corners of eye)
- On a scale of 1 to 10, grade the severity of the itching.
  Possible causes: allergies (hay fever), drug reaction, contact allergy (to makeup, lotions, etc.)

Jumping Eyelid

- How long has this been bothering you?
- Do you consume a lot of caffeine (coffee, tea, colas, chocolate)?
- Have you been having trouble sleeping?
- Are you under more stress than usual?
- Have you had injury or surgery to the eye?
  Possible causes: too much caffeine, fatigue, stress, drug reaction, Parkinson's disease, response to eye injury/pain

Lid Droop

- When did you first notice this? Has it been this way all your life?
- Is this in one eye or both?
- Are the upper lids drooping or the lower lids? Both?
- Is the lid swollen?
- Have you had cataract surgery on the drooping side?
- Have you had an eye injury?
- Does there seem to be a lump or growth in the lid?
- Do you have any type of muscular disorder?
- Do you have difficulty swallowing or chewing?
  Possible causes: birth defect, loss of muscle tone, redundant skin of upper lids, growth, injury that has damaged lid muscles, nerve paralysis, muscular dystrophy, myasthenia gravis

Light Sensitivity (Photophobia)

- When did this start?
- Is it in one eye or both?
- Do you also have eye pain? Redness? Discharge?
- Have you had any type of eye surgery?
- Have you had an injury to your eye (even years ago)?
- Are you using any type of eye drop with a red top?
- Has your vision also decreased?
  Possible causes: inflammation inside the eye, dilated pupil, drug reaction, migraine

Matter/Discharge

- When did this start?
- Are both eyes affected or just one?
- What color is the discharge (white, clear, yellow, green, bloody)?
- Are your eyes also uncomfortable? Itch? Burn? Hurt? Red?
- Have you used any eye drops or done anything else to try to clear this up? Did it help?
- Have you been exposed to someone with an eye infection?
    Possible causes: infection, allergy, dry eye

Pain

- How long has this been bothering you?
- Is it in one eye or both?
- Is the pain constant, or does it come and go?
- Does it bother you more during a certain part of the day?
- How long does the pain last?
- Does it hurt so bad that you also feel sick to your stomach?
- Do you also have a headache?
- Has your vision changed?
- Does your vision decrease when the eye is hurting?
- Describe the pain: throb, shooting, ache, gritty/sandy, sharp, dull.
- Is the eyeball or area around the eye tender to the touch?
- What seems to relieve the pain?
- Does your eye turn red when it is hurting?
- Do you use any type of eye drop? Or have you just begun using some sort of eye drop?
- Have you had eye surgery?
- Have you ever had an eye injury (even years ago)?
- Do your eyes close all the way when you sleep?
- Have you been exposed to a sun lamp, strong sun, or reflected sun (off of sand, water, or snow)?
- Have you been welding without eye protection?
    Possible causes: dry eye, foreign body, angle-closure glaucoma, drug reaction, corneal abrasion, inflammation inside the eye, eye infection, recurrent erosion syndrome, ultraviolet burn, ocular ischemia

Pressure Sensation Behind the Eyes

- When did this start?
- Is it in one eye or both?

- Do you have sinus problems?
- Have you recently had your glasses changed?
  Possible causes: sinus problems, misaligned glasses, fatigue, stress, tension, headache

Protrusion of the Eye(s)

- How long have you noticed this?
- Does only one eye seem to be pushing out or both?
- Does the protruded eye(s) seem to pulsate?
- Do you have thyroid problems?
- Do you take steroids?
- Do you take vitamin A, B, and/or D? How much?
- Is there any pain?
- Do you have sinus problems?
  Possible causes: thyroid (Graves' disease), drooping lid (lid droop of one eye can make it look as if the other eye is protruding), growth behind the eye, drug or vitamin toxicity, inflammation or infection behind the eye (as in sinus), pseudotumor of orbit

Pulling Sensation

- How long does this sensation last?
- Do both eyes seem to pull or just one?
- Does this occur with glasses on? Off? Either way?
- Do you have double vision?
- Is it constant, or does the sensation come and go?
- Have you recently had your glasses changed?
  Possible causes: misaligned glasses, incorrect glasses prescription

Rash

- When did this start?
- Have you started some new medication?
- Have you been out in the woods or doing yard work?
- Have you changed brands of eye makeup?
- Are just the lids affected or the eyes, too?
- Do you have a rash on any other part of your body?
- Describe the rash. Tiny red bumps? Blisters?
- Is there any pain?
  Possible causes: allergic reaction to drugs or chemicals, poison (ivy, oak, etc.), shingles (Herpes zoster)

Redness

- When did this start?
- Is it one eye or both?
- Is there any tearing or other discharge? What color is the discharge?
- Is there any pain or discomfort?
- Has the vision decreased?
- Is the eye sensitive to light?
- Is the eye red all over? Or is there a single blood-red patch?

If there is a blood-red patch:
- Do you have high blood pressure?
- Have you had a blow to the eye?
- Have you been straining (hard coughing or sneezing, vomiting or retching, constipation, heavy lifting, etc.)
- Do you take blood thinners or aspirin?

Possible causes: angle-closure glaucoma, iritis, eye infection, allergic reaction, dryness, hay fever, and asthma. Burst blood vessel: high blood pressure, injury, blood disorder, vitamin C deficiency

Swelling

- When did this start?
- Does it come and go?
- Is it in one eye or both?
- Are both the upper and lower lids affected?
- Is there any pain?
- Is the lid tender?
- Is the lid red and angry looking? Fevered?
- Do you feel ill?
- Is the whole lid swollen or just one area?
- Is the eyeball also red?
- Have you been using any type of eye wash, drops, or ointment?
- Have you been doing any yard work and perhaps rubbed your eyes?
- Might you have been bitten by a bug of some sort?

Possible causes: fluid retention, stye, chalazion, cellulitis, dermatochalasis, injury, allergic reaction (hay fever), contact allergy (makeup, lotions, etc.) drug reaction, malnutrition

Watery Eyes

In the Adult
- How long has this been bothering you?
- Do the tears actually stream down your cheeks?
- Are the tears clear or sticky?
- Do your eyes feel scratchy and gritty? Do they itch? Burn? Hurt?
- Do your eyes tear during any particular time of day?
- Have you been using any type of eye medication to try to clear this up? Does it help?
- Are you taking any type of antihistamine or sinus/cold/allergy medication?

    Possible causes: dry eyes, allergy, drug reaction, infection, blocked tear duct, injury

In the Infant (asked of caregiver)
- When did you first notice this?
- Is the problem in one eye or both?
- Does it come and go, or is it pretty much constant?
- Is the eye(s) also red?
- Is there a discharge? What color?
- Does the baby seem sensitive to light?
- Have you been using any medication or other treatment to try and clear this up?

    Possible causes: infection, blocked tear duct, congenital glaucoma, injury

Note: Most of the material in this chapter is taken from *The Crystal Clear Guide to Sight for Life* (Starburst Publishers) and has been reprinted with permission of the publisher.

6

Ocular Trauma-Related Questions

If the patient is a non-verbal child, you will need to rely on caregivers for the history of the trauma. However, in some cases, the adult in charge may not have witnessed the accident.

A verbal child should be questioned about the incident. Talking to the child alone (ie, without caregivers present) may give the best view on what actually happened.

Blunt Trauma

Initial Exam:
- What were you hit with?
- When did this happen?
- Did this occur on the job?
- Were you wearing protective eye wear, glasses, or contact lenses?
- Did you have an immediate loss of vision? To what extent? Did your vision return? Wholly? Partially? How long was your vision decreased?
- Were you unconscious at any time?
- Has there been any bleeding from the eye, nose, or cuts on your face?
- Are you in pain now?
- How is the vision in that eye?

- Is there a curtain over part of your vision?
- Have you seen any floaters? Flashes of light?
- Are you light sensitive?
- Are you seeing double when you look straight ahead? When you glance to the side or up and down?

Follow-up Exam:
- Have you been in any pain?
- Have you noticed any change in your vision?
- Have you noticed any curtains over your vision? Floaters? Light Flashes?
- Have you noticed any double vision? or Is your double vision any better? worse?
- Have you been light sensitive?

Bruising (Periorbital)

Initial Exam:
- What were you hit with?
- Are you in pain now?
- Does the eye itself hurt?
- Is/was the eye red?
- Did you have an immediate loss of vision? To what extent? Did your vision return? Wholly? Partially? How long was your vision decreased?
- Have you had any double vision? Numbness? Nosebleed?
- Have you used ice on the area?

Follow-up Exam:
- Has the bruising gotten any better?
- Are you still using ice packs?
- Have you had a lot of pain?
- Has the eye itself bothered you in any way? Pain? Change in vision?

Burns

Thermal

Initial Exam:
- Please describe the accident. What were you burned with?
- Were you on the job?
- Were you wearing protective eye wear or contact lenses?

- Exactly what is burned? The area around your eye, your lids, or the eye itself?
- Did you do anything right away for first aid?
- Are you in pain?
- Is the eye red?
- Did you have an immediate loss of vision? To what extent? Did your vision return? Wholly? Partially? How long was your vision decreased?

Follow-up Exam:
- Do you feel like the burn is healing?
- Have you been in any pain?
- How is your vision in that eye?
- Tell me how you've been using your eye medications.

Ultraviolet

Initial Exam:
- Please describe how this happened. Where were you? What were you doing?
- Were you on the job?
- Were you wearing protective eye wear or contact lenses?
- How long were you exposed?
- On a scale of 1 to 10, how much pain are you having?
- Have you done anything to try to relieve the pain?
- Did you have an immediate loss of vision? To what extent? Did your vision return? Wholly? Partially? How long was your vision decreased?

Follow-up Exam:
- How are your eyes feeling today?
- Have you had a lot of pain?
- How is your vision now?
- Have the eyes been red? Has there been any discharge?
- Tell me how you're using your medications.

Chemical Splash

Initial Exam:
When a patient reports with a chemical splash, initially the most important thing to find out is whether or not the eye has already been irrigated. If not (or if irrigation was not adequate), it is important to irrigate the patient immediately. You can ask some history questions while you are rinsing the eye.
- Did you irrigate the eye right after this happened? With what? For how long?

- Are you in pain?
- When did this happen?
- What were you splashed with?
- Describe the incident. Were you on the job? Was there flying debris involved?
- Were you wearing eye protection, glasses, or conatact lenses?
- Did you have an immediate loss of vision? To what extent? Did your vision return? Wholly? Partially? How long was your vision decreased?

Follow-up Exam:
- How is your eye doing today?
- Have you had a lot of pain?
- How is your vision?
- Tell me how you've been using your medications.

Foreign Body

Initial Exam:
- Is one eye involved or both?
- Any idea what got into your eye?
- Please describe the incident, if known. Did this occur on the job?
- Were you aware of any flying object hitting your eye? How hard did it hit?
- Were you wearing protective eye wear or contact lenses?
- Have you done anything to try to wash out the foreign body?
- When did your eye start hurting?
- Is the pain constant, or does it come and go?
- Did you have an immediate loss of vision? To what extent? Did your vision return? Wholly? Partially? How long was your vision decreased?

Follow-up Exam:
- How does your eye feel today? Have you had much pain?
- Have you had any more sensation of something being in your eye?
- How's your vision doing?
- Are you light sensitive?
- Has the eye been red?
- Has there been any discharge?
- Tell me how you're using your medications.

Laceration

Initial Exam:

Remember to use universal precautions for blood-borne pathogens when a patient presents with an open wound: wear gloves! When a patient comes in with a laceration of the periorbital area (not the globe) that is still bleeding, apply pressure. If there is any doubt whether or not the eyeball itself is perforated, do not apply pressure. Put a shield over the eye, and call the physician immediately.

- Please describe what happened. Were flying debris or chemicals involved? What was the nature of any debris?
- On a scale of 1 to 10, how much pain are you feeling now?
- When did the incident occur?
- Were you on the job?
- Were you wearing protective eye wear, glasses, or contact lenses?
- Did you have an immediate loss of vision? To what extent? Did your vision return? Wholly? Partially? How long was your vision decreased?
- When did you last have a tetanus shot?

Follow-up Exam:

- Does the area seem to be healing?
- Have the stitches stayed in place? (if appropriate)
- Did you get your tetanus shot? (if appropriate)
- Has there been any more bleeding?
- Has there been much swelling?
- Have you been in much pain?
- How is your vision?
- Tell me how you've been using your medications.

Exam-Prompted Questions

Sometimes, you will find things during the patient exam that the patient did not mention during the history. A patient might not complain about xanthelasma, for example, because it doesn't hurt and doesn't interfere with vision. But, it may be an important health indicator of elevated cholesterol.

This chapter consists of questions you might ask when you notice certain findings. (In some cases, I have included questions that should actually have been elicited during the patient's past medical history.) The optometric/ophthalmic assistant should remember, however, that diagnosing falls into the realm of the physician. Yet, in many cases, the assistant will recognize a condition when he or she sees it. While it would not be appropriate for the assistant to give the patient a diagnosis, it would be acceptable for the assistant to ask questions related to the probable diagnosis. Thus, the assistant who notices a cataract could *not* say, "Mrs. Cole, it looks like you have cataracts," but he or she *could* ask questions related to symptoms usually caused by cataracts.

It's beyond the scope of this book to list every finding. Many physically obvious symptoms would initially be reported by the patient. If an item isn't listed here, you might try checking Section Two of Chapter 5. Questions for follow-up exams (in which case the patient has already been diagnosed) appear in Chapter 8.

External Examination

Protruding Eye(s)

- Do you ever have any pain in either eye?
- Do you have any problems with your thyroid?
- Do you take steroids?
- Do you have sinus problems?
- Do you take vitamin A, B, and/or D? How much?

Lid Crusting

- Do your lids itch?
- Do your lids ever get red? Swollen?
- Do you have any skin problem, such as dandruff or eczema?
- Do your eyes water? Do your eyes itch? Burn?

Growths

- Have you noticed this growth before?
- Has your dermatologist or personal physician looked at it?
- How long has it been there?
- Has it grown?
- Has it changed in any way?
- Does it ever bleed? Crust over? Get sore or tender?
- Have you had similar growths?
- *Xanthelasma*: Have you had your cholesterol checked lately? What was the reading?

Ptosis

- Have you noticed that your eyelid(s) is/are drooped?
- Show me an old photograph of yourself.
- Does anyone else in your family have a drooped lid?
- Have you had any type of eye surgery?
- Have you had any type of injury to the eye or eyelid?
- Do you have myasthenia gravis?

Trichiasis

- Have you had in-turned lashes before?
- Have you had some type of eyelid surgery or injury?

Anisocoria

- Have you noticed or ever been told that your pupils aren't the same size?
- May I see an old photograph of you?
- Have you used any drops in either eye over the past several weeks?
- Has either eye ever been injured?
- Is the vision in either eye blurred?
- Do you perspire on both sides of your face?

Strabismus

Tropia

- Has your eye always turned (in/out)? If not, when did it start?
- Have you had any treatment for this problem?
- Does your vision seem to be as good in one eye as it is in the other?
- Do you ever have double vision? Are the images vertical, horizontal, or diagonal?
- Does anyone else in the family have crossed eyes?

Phoria

- Do you ever have double vision? When? Are the images vertical, horizontal, or diagonal?

Blepharochalasis

- Have you noticed this extra fold of skin over your upper lid?
- Do you get headaches?
- Do you have brow aches?
- Do your eyes ever seem like they want to close?
- Do you have any problems with your side vision?

Slit Lamp Exam

Low Tear Break-Up Time

- Do your eyes seem dry? Feel scratchy?
- Do your eyes water?
- Do your eyes ever burn?

Narrow Angles

- Do you ever have pain in either eye?
- Do you ever have headaches that center over one eye or both?

- Do one or both eyes ever get red?
- Does your vision in one or both eyes ever get hazy?
- Do you ever see halos around lights at night?

Redness

- Has this eye been bothering you in any way?
- Have you had any pain in this eye?
- Have you been rubbing this eye?
- Have you noticed any discharge from this eye?
- Did you get something in this eye recently?
    Note: If the redness appears to be a subconjunctival hemorrhage, ask the following questions:
- Do you have high blood pressure?
- Have you had a blow to the eye?
- Have you strained in any way (hard coughing or sneezing, vomiting or retching, constipation, heavy lifting, etc.)?
- Do you take blood thinners or aspirin?

Corneal Neovascularization (in the Contact Lens Wearer)

- How many hours a day are you wearing your lenses?
- Do you ever sleep in them?
- Do you ever nap in them?

Extended Wear

- Do you ever remove your lenses and leave them out overnight? How often?

Corneal Scar

- Have you ever had any injury to this eye, even years ago?
- How is your vision in this eye?
- Do you have problems with glare from lights?
- Do you ever see halos around lights at night?

Corneal Rust Ring

- Do you remember ever getting a piece of metal in this eye?
- When?
- What were you doing when it got in there?
- Was the particle traveling under force?
- Did you go to the doctor to have it removed?

Pterygium

- Had you noticed this little growth on your eye before?
- Have any of your doctors commented on it?
- How long has it been there?
- Does it seem to be growing at all?
- Do you work outside or in a dusty environment?

Cataract

Nuclear Sclerotic

- How is your vision?
- Do you feel you see as well now as you did 5 years ago?
- Do you see as well out of one eye as the other?
- Do you wear glasses to read? Can you read without them? Is this something new?
- Have you noticed any change in your color vision?
- Has there been any change in your depth perception?
- Do you have any problems with glare?
- Do you see halos around lights at night?

Posterior Subcapsular

- Do you have any problems seeing in bright light?
- Do you have any problems seeing at night when car lights hit you?

Capsule Opacity

- Do you think that your vision is as clear now as when you first had your cataract removed?
- Are you having any problems with your vision due to glare?

Ocular Disorder-Related Questions for Follow-up Exams

The questions in this chapter are to be used at follow-up exams when the physician has previously given a diagnosis. In some cases, you are referred to another chapter for the appropriate material.

When doing a history on a patient as a follow-up of a specific problem, you should describe the patient's evaluation of his or her own status (stable, improving, worsening) as well as make a note of any new symptoms that the patient has described. "Patient has no complaints" is *never* an adequate history for a follow-up exam.

Following several questions is material in parentheses. The parenthetical notes are to indicate the possible cause of that group of symptoms in an affected individual. This is included to help you understand why a particular question (or set of questions) is important. In addition, certain questions may be repeated because they are part of a cluster of symptoms found in a certain ocular disorder. Obviously, there is no need to ask the patient the same question twice; the material is repeated so that you can learn the symptom clusters.

External Adnexa

Blepharitis

- How do your lids seem to be doing?
- How often are you using your drops/ointment?
- Are you still scrubbing your lids? Tell me how you do that, and how often.
- Rate the following as not a problem, improved, same, or worse: crusting, itching, redness of lid margin.
- Are you experiencing any of the following: scratchiness, stinging, excessive watering, dandruff.

Blepharochalasis

- Do you think that the lid droop is any better, the same, or worse since your last visit?
- Have you noticed any change in your side vision?

Blepharospasm

- Do you think that the lid twitch is better, the same, or worse?
- About how much of the following do you use each day: soft drinks (with caffeine), tea, coffee, chocolate, stimulants such as Vivarin (SmithKline Beecham, Philadelphia).
- On a scale of 1 to 5, rate your stress level, with 0 being no stress and 5 being the most stress.
- About how much sleep do you get each night? Is this pretty much uninterrupted, or do you awaken often during the night?

Skin Cancer

- Did you have one or more severe sunburns during childhood or adolescence?
- Did you or do you work in a job with a lot of exposure to the sun?
- Do you tend to sunburn easily?
- Have you noticed any new growths? How long have they been there? Have they grown?
- Have you noticed any change in any old moles or growths, such as changes in color, shape, or size?
- Do any growths tend to bleed, crust over, then bleed again without completely healing?
- If a growth was previously removed, is there any sign that it may be recurring?

Cellulitis

- Are you still using your medications?
- How are you feeling? Have you had any fever?
- Tell me if the following are better, worse, or unchanged: lid swelling, lid redness, fever in the lid, lid tenderness, pain.

Contact Dermatitis

- Is the rash better, worse, or the same? Has it spread?
- Is there any pain or other discomfort? Does it itch? Ooze?
- Have you stopped wearing makeup and/or using face creams and lotions as directed?
- Do you have any idea what might have caused the rash?
- Tell me how you're using your medication(s).

Ectropion

- Are your eyes watering a lot?
- Do your eyes feel sandy or gritty?
- Do your eyes itch and burn?
- How is your vision?
- Are you using artificial tears? How often?

Entropion

- Do your eyes feel scratchy or as if there's something in them? Is this constant, or does it come and go?
- Do your eyes water a lot?
- How is your vision?

Growths

Chalazion/Stye
- Has the swelling gone down any?
- Has it drained at all?
- Is the area sore or tender?
- How is your vision?
- Are you using your drops/ointment? Hot packs?

Moles and Other Lesions
- Have you noticed any change in size, shape, or color since your last visit?
- Has the area been raw, bled, or scabbed over?
- Have any more lesions appeared? Where?

Note: If the patient has had a lesion excised, see the postoperative questions in the plastics section in Chapter 9.

Xanthelasma

- Have you noticed any change in the size of the growths?
- How is your cholesterol level?

Herpes Zoster

- Are the sores beginning to clear up at all?
- Have new ulcers appeared anywhere?
- Are you having a lot of pain?
- How is your vision?
- Is your eye uncomfortable in any way?
- Are you light sensitive?
- Please tell me how you are using your medications.

Ptosis

- Has your lid position changed any since you were here last?
- Have your pupils seemed to be the same size?
- Do you feel that the lid is covering up or cutting off part of your vision?
- Have you experienced any double vision?
- Have you noticed any unusual fatigue?
- Have you experienced any trouble swallowing or chewing?

Trichiasis

- Do your eyes feel scratchy or as if there's something in them?
- Is there any discharge?
- Can you see any in-grown lashes when you look in the mirror? Have you tried to pull them out yourself?
- How is your vision?

Lacrimal

Dacryocystitis

- How are you feeling in general? Have you had a fever?
- Tell me if the following are improved, unimproved, or about the same: pain, swelling, redness.
- Tell me how you're taking your medications.
- Are you using hot packs? How often?

Dry Eye

- Have your eyes been watering? When does this seem to be the worst?
- What seems to aggravate your eyes the most?
- Do your eyes feel scratchy? Do they itch? Burn?
- What brand of artificial tears are you using? How often? Do they seem to help?
- Are you using an artificial tear ointment at night? What brand?
   Note: Also ask about any other related treatments, such as vitamin therapy, use of a humidifier, lid scrubs, etc.

Nasolacrimal Obstruction

- Is the tearing better? Worse? The same?
- Is there any crusting or matter in the eye?
- Tell me about your eye medications.
- Are you massaging the area? How often?

External Eye

Conjunctivitis

- Do you feel that the problem is getting better?
- Is there any discharge now? How much? When does it appear? What color is it?
- Is the redness any better? Worse? The same?
- How does the eye feel? Is there any itching? Burning? Pain? Feeling as if there is something in the eye?
- How is your vision?
- Are you sensitive to light?
- Has anyone else in the family developed the problem since you were here last?
- Tell me how you are using your medications.

Episcleritis

- Are you having any pain now?
- Is the redness better, worse, or the same?
- Is your eye watering much?
- Are you sensitive to light?
- How is your vision?
- Have you noticed any halos around lights?
- Tell me how you are using your medications.

Exophthalmos

- Have you noticed any change in your eye(s) or lids?
- Is your eye ever uncomfortable? Does it ever feel scratchy or as if something is in it?
- Are you having any problem with tearing?
- Do your eyes ever burn?
- Are you using artificial tears? What brand? How often?
- Do you use artificial tear ointment at night? What brand?
- Have you had any double vision?
- Have you had your thyroid checked since you were here last?

Growths

Conjunctival Cyst or Pingueculum
- Has it changed in size since your last visit?
- Does it ever get red? Irritated?

Pterygium
- Do you feel that the pterygium has grown any since your last visit?
- Has your vision changed in that eye?
- Does it ever get red? Irritated?
- Are you wearing lenses with UV protection whenever you are outdoors?

Scleritis

- Do you feel that the condition is better, worse, or the same?
- Are you having any pain? Is the eyeball still tender?
- Has the redness decreased at all?
- Has the eye been watering?
- Has there been any swelling around the eye?
- Are you light sensitive?
- Does the eye seem resistant to movement?
- How is your vision? Any change at all?
- *If appropriate*: Did you have the lab work done as the doctor requested?
- Tell me how you are using your medications.

Cornea

Abrasion

- How does your eye feel today? Does the eye still feel scratchy or as if there is still something in it? Are you having any pain?
- Do you ever awaken at night or in the morning and your lid seems stuck to your eye?
- How is your vision?
- Are you light sensitive?
- Has the eye been red?
- Has there been any discharge?
- Tell me how you're using your medications.

Dystrophy

- How is your vision?
- Do you see halos around lights?
- Do you have any discomfort, such as scratchiness or feeling like there is something in your eye?
- Are you using any eye drops? Tell me how you use them.

Edema

- How is your vision doing? Has it cleared up at all?
- Do you have episodes of blurriness? At what time of day?
- Do you notice colored halos around lights?
- Are your eyes uncomfortable in any way? Painful?
- *If appropriate*: Are you still wearing your contacts? How long has it been since you wore them? Or, How many hours a day are you wearing them?
- Tell me how you are using your medications.

Exposure Keratitis

- Are your eyes uncomfortable in any way? Are you experiencing any pain? Do the eyes ever burn? Feel scratchy?
- Do your eyes water?
- How is your vision doing? Has it changed?
- Are you using artificial tears and/or ointment? What brand? How often?
- *If appropriate*: Are you taping or patching your eye(s) shut at night? Do you feel that the eye stays closed?

Infective Keratitis

- Do you feel that the problem is getting better?
- Is there any discharge? How much? When does it appear? What color is it?
- Is there any redness?
- How does the eye feel? Is there any itching? Burning? Pain? Feeling as if there is something in the eye?
- How is your vision?
- Are you sensitive to light?
- Has anyone else in the family developed the problem since you were here last?
- Tell me how you are using your medications.

Keratoconus

- How is your vision? Has it changed since your last visit?
- Have you experienced any gradually decreased vision? Change in your color vision? Change in depth perception? Halos around lights at night? Glare from lights? Double vision? Light sensitivity? (cataracts)
- Have your eyes been bothering you at all? Itching? Matter? Crusting?
- Do you find yourself rubbing your eyes a lot?
- If appropriate, ask questions for a contact lens follow-up exam (see Chapter 2). Pay special attention to questions related to the lens fit.

Recurrent Erosion Syndrome

- How does your eye feel now? Are you having any pain? Scratchiness? The sensation that something is in your eye?
- Do you awaken at night or in the morning with pain?
- Do you awaken at night or in the morning and your lid is stuck to your eye?
- Are you experiencing any light sensitivity?
- How is your vision? Has it changed since your last visit?
- Tell me how you are using your medications.

Cataract

- How is your vision holding up?
- Are you able to see to drive?
- Are you able to see to perform your work on the job?
- Are you able to see to do things around the house?
- Are you able to see to do your hobbies?
- Can you see to read and handle your personal business?
- Have you given up any activities because of your vision?

- What is the one thing you can't do because of the cataracts that you would like to be able to do?
- Have you noticed any change in your color vision? Have others told you that your clothes don't match or complain when you adjust the color on the television set?
- Have you noticed any change in your depth perception?
- Have you noticed that objects seem one size with one eye and larger or smaller with the other?
- Does one eye see better than the other? If yes, has the weaker eye always been weaker?
- Are you bothered by glare from the sun during the day or from car headlights at night?
- Do you see halos around lights at night?
- What bothers you most about your vision/eyes?

Open-Angle Glaucoma

- How is your vision? Do you feel like it has changed?
- Have you had any discomfort in either eye?
- Show me your eye medications (drops and pills). How often are you taking each one? When did you last use each one?
- Are you faithful about using your medications as directed, day in and day out?

Note: If the patient was put on a new medication, you should also ask:

- How are you doing with the new drops/pills? Any problems?
- Have you noticed any changes in your health or how you feel?
- Have you experienced any decreased appetite? Nausea? Stomach upset? Headaches? Insomnia? Heart palpitations? Anything else unusual?

Internal Inflammations and Retina

Diabetic Retinopathy

See the section on diabetes in Chapter 4.

Hypertensive Retinopathy

See the section on hypertension in Chapter 4.

Hyphema

- Is your eye uncomfortable in any way? Painful?
- How is your vision? Any change since last visit?

- Are you sensitive to light?
- Have you been keeping your head elevated when you lie down?
- Have you been avoiding strenuous activities?
   Note: Hyphema is usually accompanied by other results of trauma. Be sure to ask history questions about them as well.

Iritis

- Is your eye still painful? Is it better, worse, or the same as your last visit?
- Has the redness improved at all?
- Are you still sensitive to light? Is it any better than when you were here last?
- How is your vision?
- Tell me how you are using your eye drops.

Ischemic Optic Neuropathy

- How has your vision been? Any episodes where the vision goes out then returns?
- Does the other eye seem to be affected?
- Have you been having any headaches? (If yes, follow with headache history as in Chapter 5.)
- Do you have any tenderness in the temples?
- Have you noticed any other discomfort? Pain?
- *If appropriate:* Have you had the lab work done that the doctor requested?
- Tell me about your medications.

Macular Degeneration

- Has there been any change in your vision since your last visit?
- Are you looking at your Amsler grid regularly? Have you noticed any changes on it?
- Has there been any change in what you are able to do because of your vision?
- When must you renew your drivers' license?
- *If appropriate:* Are you taking the vitamins that the doctor recommended?

Optic Neuritis

- How is your vision? Does it seem to fluctuate?
- Are there any blind spots in your vision? Is that better or worse than when you were here last?
- How is your side vision doing?

- Are you having any problems with depth perception? Color vision?
- Has your eye been uncomfortable in any way? Sore? Achy?
- *If appropriate*: Have you had the lab work that the doctor requested?
- *If appropriate*: Tell me how you are using your medications.

Papilledema

- How is your vision? Any episodes where the vision blurs or blacks out? How long does that last?
- Have you experienced any double vision? Or, Is your double vision any better since your last visit?
- Are you having any headaches? (If yes, follow with headache history as in Chapter 5.)
- Tell me about your medications.

Papillitis

The two types of papillitis are ischemic optic neuropathy and optic neuritis. Please refer to those specific headings for appropriate history questions.

Posterior Vitreous Detachment

- Has there been any change in your vision?
- Have the floaters changed in any way? Increased? Decreased? Different shapes?
- Have you experienced any further light flashes? Do these seem to be increasing or decreasing in occurrence?
- Have you experienced a film or curtain over your vision?

Retinal Detachment

Presumably, any retinal detachment would be repaired once it is discovered. Please see Chapter 9 for appropriate postoperative questions.

Retinal/Vitreous Hemorrhage

- How is your vision doing? Has there been any improvement or worsening?
- Are you seeing "floaters"? Has this changed since your last visit? Fewer or more of them? Larger or smaller?
- Have you experienced any episode of light flashes?
- Have you noticed a curtain or veil over part of your vision?
- Have you had any pain?
- *If appropriate*: Have you been keeping your head elevated?

Toxoplasmosis

- Have you experienced any light flashes? Floaters? Blurred vision? Loss of side vision? Loss of central vision? (retinitis)
- Have you experienced any generalized vision loss? A loss of peripheral vision? (papillitis)
- Have you experienced any gradually decreased vision? Change in your color vision? Change in depth perception? Halos around lights at night? Glare from lights? Double vision? Light sensitivity? (cataracts)
- Have you experienced a sudden vision loss? Vision loss that comes and goes? Decreased depth perception? Change in color vision? Pain? Loss of central vision? (optic neuritis)
- Have you experienced redness? Pain? Light sensitivity? Tearing? Blurred vision? (iritis)
- Have you experienced any pain? Redness? Light sensitivity? Blurred vision? (uveitis)

Uveitis

- Is your vision better, worse, or the same compared to the last visit?
- Have you experienced any distortion in your vision?
- Have you experienced any floaters or light flashes?
- Have you noticed a veil or curtain over your vision?
- Do you see halos around lights?
- Has your eye been uncomfortable in any way?
- Has the eye been red? Is this better, worse, or the same?
- Are you sensitive to light?
- Tell me how you are using your medications.

Muscles/Nerves

Nerve Palsies (listed in alphabetical order)

Bell's (Seventh)

- Do you think that the muscle weakness has improved any since you were here last?
- Are you able to move your mouth on that side? Blink?
- Are you having any trouble eating? Do you find that you drool?
- Is your eye uncomfortable in any way? Does it ever burn? Feel scratchy?
- Does your eye water?
- How is your vision? Has it changed?

- Are you using artificial tears and/or ointment? What brand? How often?
- *If appropriate*: Are you taping or patching your eye shut at night? Do you feel that the eye stays closed?

Fourth or Sixth

- How is your vision?
- How is the double vision? Is that better or worse since your last visit? Are you covering or closing one eye to eliminate the second image?
- *If appropriate*: Does the prism in your glasses seem to help?

Third

- How is your vision?
- Any problems seeing up close with that eye? Is this any better than when you were here last?
- Has your vision been doubled? Is that better or worse since your last visit? Are you covering or closing one eye to eliminate the second image?
- Do you feel that the eyelid is lower or higher than when you were here last?
- *If appropriate*: Does the prism in your glasses seem to help?

Strabismus

Notes: If strabismus has been corrected surgically, see postoperative questions in Chapter 9. If strabismus is due to a nerve palsy in an adult, see section on nerve palsies, above. If this is a strabismus follow-up on a child, see below. (If diagnosis also includes amblyopia, see section on amblyopia, later in this chapter.)

Ask the caregiver:

- Do you still notice the eye(s) crossing? Which eye? In or out?
- Does the eye cross all the time or just sometimes? When?
- Would you say that the crossing is better, worse, or the same as your last visit?

If appropriate: ask the following questions:

- Is he or she wearing the glasses?
- About how many hours a day does he or she wear them?
- Do the eyes seem to cross when the glasses are on? How about when he or she takes them off?
- Does he or she tend to look over the glasses or through them?
- Does he or she look through or over the bifocal when looking at up-close things?

Refractive Conditions

Amblyopia

Granted, amblyopia is not always refractive in cause. Remember, treating amblyopia is done in childhood, so most of your questions will be asked of a caregiver.

- Are you using a patch? Over which eye?
- About how many hours a day does the child actually wear the patch?
- Are you having problems getting him or her to wear the patch or to leave it on?
- How does he or she seem to be doing, visually, when the patch is on? Any problems with school work? Getting around the neighborhood? Seeing the television?
- Does either eye cross when you take the patch off?
- *If appropriate*: Is he or she wearing the glasses all the time? If not, about how many hours a day? Does he or she seem to look over the glasses a lot, or is he or she actually looking through them?

Aphakia

- Do you wear lenses with UV protection when you go outdoors?
- Have you noticed any floaters or light flashes?
- Have you ever noticed a curtain or veil over part of your vision?

If the patient wears spectacles, ask the following questions:

- How are your glasses doing for you?
- Are you able to see what you need to see?
- Can you see better if you move your glasses a bit?
- Are you able to see to read?
- Do you have any double vision?
- Do you have problems judging distances?
- Do the frames hurt your nose or behind your ears?
- *If appropriate*: Have you had any problems adjusting to your new glasses?
- *If appropriate*: ask questions about his or her contact lenses (see Chapter 2). Pay special attention to questions that would indicate contact lens intolerance.

Hyperopia

- How is your vision at a distance? Up close?
- Are your glasses doing the job for you?

- Do you wear your glasses all the time? If not, when? For what activities?
- Do you ever have episodes of eye pain? Redness? Blurred vision? Do you ever see halos around lights? (angle-closure glaucoma)
- *If appropriate*: Have you had any problems adjusting to your new glasses?

Myopia

- How is your vision at a distance? Up close?
- Are your glasses doing the job for you?
- Do you wear your glasses all the time? If not, when? For what activities?
- Have you noticed any floaters? Light flashes? A curtain over part of your vision? (posterior vitreous detachment; retinal detachment)
- *If appropriate*: Have you had any problems adjusting to your new glasses?

Presbyopia

- How is your close-up vision?
- Are you wearing your glasses to read? Does taking your glasses off make your reading more clear?
- Show me where you hold your reading material.
- Are you having to hold material closer than you would like to?
- Do you find yourself holding material farther away in order to see it more clearly?
- Are you having any problems seeing middle distances, such as the computer screen or items on shelves?
- Have you noticed any double vision or split vision?
- *If appropriate*: Have you had any problems adjusting to your new glasses?

Postoperative Questions

Plastics

- Have you been uncomfortable?
- Have you had any pain?
- How is your vision?
- Do you feel that the area has been healing well?
- Has there been any swelling? Bruising? Bleeding? Redness? Have these decreased?
- Is the area hot or tender?
- Have the wounds been oozing at all?
- Have any of the stitches come out?
- Have your eyes been watering? Burning? Stinging?
- Have you been using the ice/hot packs?
- Tell me how you've been using your medications.

   Note: If the plastic surgery was for removal of a lesion, on follow-up exams it is pertinent to ask the patient if he or she has noticed any regrowth or recurrence.

Enucleation

- Have you had much discomfort?
- Have you had any pain?
- Has there been a lot of swelling? Bruising? Redness? Have these decreased?
- Is the area hot or tender?
- Has there been a discharge?
- Has the conformer stayed in place?
- How is the vision in your other eye?
- How is your depth perception? Are you learning to judge distances?
- Have your family or friends been supportive?
- Tell me how you've been using your medications.

Strabismus Repair

- Have you been very uncomfortable?
- Have you had any pain?
- Has there been a lot of swelling? Bruising? Redness? Have these decreased?
- Has there been a discharge?
- Has your eye been feeling scratchy, as if there's something in it?
- How is your vision?
- Have you been seeing double?
- Do you feel that your eyes are holding straight? That they are working together?
- Tell me how you've been using your medications.

Corneal Transplant

- Have you had much discomfort?
- Have you had any pain?
- Does your eye feel scratchy?
- Has there been a lot of swelling? Bruising? Redness? Have these decreased?
- Has there been any discharge? Tearing?
- How is your vision? Does it fluctuate from day to day? How? Does it fluctuate during the day? Please describe this.
- Have you experienced any double vision? Distortion?
- Are you sensitive to light? Do you have problems with glare? Do you see halos around lights?
- Tell me how you're using your medications.

Refractive Surgery

- Is your eye uncomfortable in any way? Scratchy feeling?
- Have you had any pain?
- Has there been much redness?
- Has there been any discharge? Tearing?
- How is your vision? Does it fluctuate from one day to the next? How? Does it fluctuate during the day? Describe this. Is it more clear when you get up in the morning, or does it progressively clear as the day goes by? Do you see equally well at distance as you do up close?
- Have you experienced any double vision? Distortion?
- Are you light sensitive? Have problems with glare? See halos around lights?
- Tell me how you're using your medications.
- *If appropriate*: Has the contact lens stayed on your eye?

Surgical Trabeculectomy

- Have you had much discomfort?
- Have you had any pain?
- Does your eye feel scratchy? Have you noticed any sensation of fullness?
- Has there been a lot of swelling? Bruising? Redness? Have these decreased?
- Has there been any discharge? Bleeding? Tearing?
- Are you sensitive to light?
- How is your vision?
- Have you noticed any light flashes or floaters?
- Tell me how you're using your medications.

Laser Trabeculectomy

- Have you had any discomfort? Scratchiness?
- Have you had any pain?
- Has there been any redness?
- How is your vision?
- Are you sensitive to light?
- Have you noticed any light flashes or floaters? Halos around lights? Areas of missing or distorted vision?
- Tell me how you're using your medications.

Laser Iridotomy

- How is your eye? Have you had any discomfort? Scratchiness?
- Have you had any pain?
- Has your eye been red?
- How is your vision?
- Are you sensitive to light?
- Have you noticed any light flashes or floaters? Halos around lights? Areas of missing or distorted vision?
- Tell me how you're using your medications.

Cataract Extraction

Postoperative Day 1

- How is your eye feeling?
- Have you had any discomfort? Itching?
- Have you had any pain?
- Did everyone treat you well at the hospital/surgical center?
- Did you sleep well last night?
- *If appropriate*: How is your vision? Have you taken the patch off at all? Tell me how you are using your medications.

Subsequent Postoperative Visits

- How is your eye?
- Have you had any pain?
- How is your vision? Does it seem to fluctuate at all? Do your glasses make it better or worse?
- Have you had any double vision?
- Have you noticed any problem with glare?
- Have you noticed any floaters or light flashes?
- Have you had any discomfort? Scratchiness? Tenderness? Light sensitivity? Redness? Discharge?
- Has your eyelid been swollen or drooped?
- Tell me how you are using your medications.

Laser Capsulotomy

- How is your eye? Have you had any discomfort? Scratchiness?
- Have you had any pain?

- Has your eye been red?
- How is your vision?
- Are you sensitive to light?
- Have you noticed any light flashes or floaters?
- Tell me how you're using your medications.

Retinal Laser

- Have you had any discomfort? Scratchiness?
- Have you had any pain?
- Has your eye been red?
- How is your vision?
- Have you noticed any distortions in your vision? Missing areas of vision? Changes in your peripheral vision? Changes in your night vision?
- Are you sensitive to light?
- Have you noticed any light flashes or floaters?
- Tell me how you're using your medications.
  Note: Also, be sure to ask the patient relevant questions about the condition that called for treatment (i.e., hypertension, diabetes, etc.).

Retinal Detachment Repair

- Have you had much discomfort? Does your eye feel scratchy?
- Have you had any pain?
- Has there been a lot of swelling? Bruising? Redness? Have these decreased?
- Has there been any discharge? Tearing?
- Are you sensitive to light?
- How is your vision?
- Have you noticed any light flashes, floaters, or curtains? Any missing or distorted areas of vision? Any double vision?
- Tell me how you're using your medications.

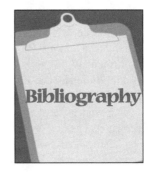

Bibliography

Bibliography

American Medical Association/Health Care Financing Administration. *Guidelines for Evaluation and Management Services.* May 1997.

Asbell RL. *New Single-Organ-System Guidelines for Eye Examinations.* ASCRS website: www.ascrs.org/publications/ao/6_4_52.html; access date 5/19/98.

Bloch RS, Henkind P. Ocular manifestations of endocrine and metabolic diseases. In: Tasman W, Jaeger EA, eds. *Duane's Ophthalmology on CD-ROM.* Philadelphia, PA: Lippincott-Raven Publishers; 1996.

Billings JA, Stoeckle JD. *The Clinical Encounter: A Guide to the Medical Interview and Case Presentation.* St. Louis, MO: Mosby-Year Book, Inc.; 1989.

Brown B. *The Low Vision Handbook.* Thorofare, NJ: SLACK Incorporated.; 1997.

Cassin G, ed. *Fundamentals for Ophthalmic Technical Personnel.* Philadelphia: W.B. Saunders; 1995.

Complete Drug Reference, 1997 ed. Yonkers, NY: Consumer Reports Books; 1997.

Documentation in Depth: A Comprehensive Guide for Physicians. St. Paul, MN: Medical Learning, Inc.; 1997.

Duvall B, Kershner RM. *Ophthalmic Medications and Pharmacology.* Thorofare, NJ: SLACK Incorporated; 1998.

Forster RK. Endophthalmitis. In: Tasman W, Jaeger EA, eds. *Duane's Ophthalmology on CD-ROM.* Philadelphia: Lippincott-Raven Publishers; 1996.

Foster CS. Syphilis. In: Tasman W, Jaeger EA, eds. *Duane's Ophthalmology on CD-ROM.* Philadelphia: Lippincott-Raven Publishers; 1996.

Frangieh GT, Lee JS, Smith RE. The cornea in systemic disease. In: Tasman W, Jaeger EA, eds. *Duane's Ophthalmology on CD-ROM.* Philadelphia: Lippincott-Raven Publishers; 1996.

Frayer WC, Scheie HG. Cataract surgery. In: Duane TD, ed. *Clinical Ophthalmology.* Philadelphia: Harper & Row; 1984.

Gayton JL, Bittinger MD. How we fixed our coding problem... *Ophthalmology Management.* 1998;24(1):26-29.

Gayton JL, Ledford JR. *The Crystal Clear Guide to Sight for Life: A Complete Manual of Eye Care for Those Over 40.* Lancaster, PA: Starburst Publishers; 1996.

Godfrey WA. Acute Anterior Uveitis. In: Tasman W, Jaeger EA, eds. *Duane's Ophthalmology on CD-ROM.* Philadelphia, PA: Lippincott-Raven Publishers; 1996.

Goldbert MR. Sickle cell retinopathy. In: Tasman W, Jaeger EA, eds. *Duane's Ophthalmology on CD-ROM.* Philadelphia, PA: Lippincott-Raven Publishers; 1996.

Griffith HW. *Complete Guide to Prescription and Non-Prescription Drugs,* 1998 ed. New York, NY: Berkley Publishing Group; 1998.

Gross J, Gross FJ, Friedman AH. Systemic infections and inflammatory diseases. In: Tasman W, Jaeger EA, eds. *Duane's Ophthalmology on CD-ROM.* Philadelphia: Lippincott-Raven Publishers; 1996.

Hansen VC. *Ocular Motility.* Thorofare, NJ: SLACK Incorporated; 1988.

Hetherington J Jr. Classification and examination. In: Duane TD, ed. *Clinical Ophthalmology.* Philadelphia: Harper & Row; 1984.

Kornmehl EW. Lyme disease. In: Tasman W, Jaeger EA, eds. *Duane's Ophthalmology on CD-ROM.* Philadelphia: Lippincott-Raven Publishers; 1996.

Ledford JK. Cracking the history of pain. *Professional Medical Assistant.* 1994;27(1):21-22.

Ledford JK. *Exercises in Refractometry.* Thorofare, NJ: SLACK Incorporated; 1990.

Ledford JK. *In-Office Training Manual and Series Review.* Thorofare, NJ: SLACK Incorporated; 1992.

Pavan-Langston D. *Manual of Ocular Diagnosis and Therapy*, 2nd ed. Boston, MA: Little, Brown and Co. 1985.

Physicians' Desk Reference, 52nd ed. Montvale, NJ: Medical Economics Company; 1998.

Physicians' Desk Reference for Nonprescription Drugs, 19th ed. Montvale, NJ: Medical Economics Company; 1998.

Pickett K. *Overview of Ocular Surgery and Surgical Counseling*. Thorofare, NJ: SLACK Incorporated; 1999.

Raakow PL. *Contact Lenses*. Thorofare, NJ: SLACK Incorporated; 1988.

Rogers GL, Bremer DL, McGregor ML. Pediatric Ocular Trauma. In: Tasman W, Jaeger EA, eds. *Duane's Ophthalmology on CD-ROM*. Philadelphia: Lippincott-Raven Publishers; 1996.

Sanborn GE, Magargal LE. Arterial obstructive disease of the eye. In: Tasman W, Jaeger EA, eds. *Duane's Ophthalmology on CD-ROM*. Philadelphia: Lippincott-Raven Publishers; 1996.

Sivalingam A, Bolling J, Goldberg RE, Sivalingam J, Magargal LE. Ocular abnormalities in acquired heart disease. In: Tasman W, Jaeger EA, eds. *Duane's Ophthalmology on CD-ROM*. Philadelphia: Lippincott-Raven Publishers; 1996.

Stephens GL, Davis JK. Spectacle Lenses. In: Tasman W, Jaeger EA, eds. *Duane's Ophthalmology on CD-ROM*. Philadelphia: Lippincott-Raven Publishers; 1996.

Tabbara KF. Toxoplasmosis. In: Tasman W, Jaeger EA, eds. *Duane's Ophthalmology on CD-ROM*. Philadelphia: Lippincott-Raven Publishers; 1996.

Traboulsi EI, Green WR, O'Donnell FE Jr. Clinical Manifestations of Albinism. In: Tasman W, Jaeger EA, eds. *Duane's Ophthalmology on CD-ROM*. Philadelphia: Lippincott-Raven Publishers; 1996.

VanBoemel GB. *Functional Visual Loss: How to evaluate the "difficult" patient*. Lecture.

Vaughan DG, Asbury T, Riordan-Eva P. *General Ophthalmology*, 13th ed. Norwalk, CT: Appleton & Lange; 1992.

Wang FM. Perinatal ophthalmology. In: Tasman W, Jaeger EA, eds. *Duane's Ophthalmology on CD-ROM*. Philadelphia: Lippincott-Raven Publishers; 1996.

Woodworth KE, Campbell RC, Dean CA, DuBois LG, Ledford JK. Analysis of tasks performed by certified ophthalmic medical personnel. *Ophthalmology*. 1995;102(12):1973-1986.

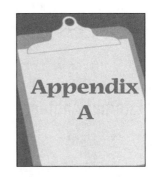

Appendix
A

Appendix A
Common Ophthalmic
Abbreviations

This list of ophthalmic abbreviations is intended as a guide during history taking. For the list to be most serviceable, you will need to customize it by adding those abbreviations used in your particular office.

Ocular Anatomy

External Anatomy

R—right
L—left
OD—right eye
OS—left eye
OU—both eyes
UL—upper lid
LL—lower lid
ULOU—upper lids, both eyes
LLOU—lower lids, both eyes
RUL—right upper lid
LUL—left upper lid
RLL—right lower lid
LLL—left lower lid

Anatomy of the Globe

conj—conjunctiva
K—cornea
—angle
P—pupil
A/C—anterior chamber
aq—aqueous
P/C—posterior chamber
vit—vitreous
ret—retina
RPE—retinal pigment epithelium
ON—optic nerve

Exam Types/Appointments

ADPL—average daily patient load
CEE—complete eye exam
FUV—follow-up visit
NS—no show
OV—office visit

Re—recheck
RTO—return to office
RTC—return to clinic
RV—return visit

History

Descriptions

pt—patient
DOB—date of birth
m—male
f—female
yo—year old
mo—month old
w—white (Caucasian)
b—black (African American)
o—Oriental
i—Indian (Native American or person from India)

Basic Terms

<—less (smaller) than
>—greater (larger) than
↑—increase
↓—decrease
Δ—change
CC—chief complaint
c/o—complains of
DOS—date of surgery
FH/FHx—family history
HPI—history of present illness
Hx—history
meds—medication
NKA—no known allergies
NKDA—no known drug allergies
PFSH—past, family, social history
PH/PHx—past history
PI—present illness
P/O—postoperative
ROS—review of systems
Rx—prescription, prescribed, medication
S/P—status post
Sx—symptoms

Diseases/Conditions

AIDS—acquired immune deficiency syndrome
AODM—adult-onset diabetes mellitus
BCC—basal cell carcinoma
CA—cancer/carcinoma
CHF—congestive heart failure
CN—cranial nerve
CNS—central nervous system
COPD—chronic obstructive pulmonary disease
CP—cerebral palsy
CVA—cerebrovascular accident (stroke)
CVD—cardiovascular disease
DI—diabetes insipidus
DM—diabetes mellitus
FB—foreign body
HBP—high blood pressure
IDDM—insulin-dependent diabetes mellitus
JODM—juvenile-onset diabetes mellitus
JRA—juvenile rheumatoid arthritis
MD—muscular dystrophy
MI—myocardial infarction
MR—mentally retarded
MS—multiple sclerosis
NIDDM—non-insulin-dependent diabetes mellitus
RA—rheumatoid arthritis
RF—rheumatic fever
SLE—systemic lupus erythematosus
STD—sexually transmitted disease
TB—tuberculosis
VD—venereal disease

Miscellaneous

BS—blood sugar
ETOH—alcohol
HA—headache
HOH—hard of hearing
N&V—nausea and vomiting
ROS—review of systems
SOB—shortness of breath

Visual Acuity

VA—visual acuity
DA—distant acuity
NA—near acuity
Cc—with correction
Sc—without correction

Spectacles/lenses

gl—glasses
add—addition (as in bifocal or trifocal)
segs—segments
BF/bi—bifocal
TF/tri—trifocal

Contact Lenses

Types/Materials

CAB—cellulose acetate butyrate
DSCL—disposable soft contact lens
DW—daily wear
EW—extended wear
EWCL—extended wear contact lens
GPCL (or GP)—gas permeable contact lens
HCL—hard contact lens
HEMA—hydroxyethylmethacrylate
PMMA—polymethylmethacrylate
SCL—soft contact lens
TBC—therapeutic bandage contact

Lens Problems

GPC—giant papillary conjunctivitis
OWS—over-wear syndrome
TLS—tight-lens syndrome

Notations

Dx—diagnosis
R/O—rule out
Tx—treatment
WNL—within normal limits

Glaucoma

COAG—chronic open-angle glaucoma
CSG—chronic simple glaucoma
NAG—narrow-angle glaucoma

Lens

cat—cataract
IOL—intraocular lens
NS—nuclear sclerosis
PSC—posterior subcapsular cataract

Retina/Vitreous

ARMD—age-related macular degeneration
BDR—background diabetic retinopathy
BVO—branch vein occlusion
CME—cystoid macular edema
CRAO—central retinal artery occlusion
CRVO—central retinal vein occlusion
CSR—central serous retinopathy
DR—diabetic retinopathy
ERM—epiretinal membrane
ION—ischemic optic neuropathy
MD—macular degeneration
NPDR—non-proliferative diabetic retinopathy
ON—optic neuritis
PDR—proliferative diabetic retinopathy
POA—primary optic atrophy
POHS—presumed ocular histoplasmosis syndrome
PVD—posterior vitreous detachment
RD—retinal detachment
RLF—retrolental fibroplasia
SMD—senile macular degeneration
VH—vitreous hemorrhage

Surgery/Treatment

2° IOL—secondary intraocular lens implant
ALPC—argon laser photocoagulation
ALT—argon laser trabeculoplasty
DCR—dacryocystorhinostomy

ECCE—extracapsular cataract extraction
FS—fascenella-servat
I&D—incision & drainage
IOL—intraocular lens
ICCE—intracapsular cataract extraction
NCB—noncosmetic blepharoplasty
PI—peripheral iridectomy
PKP—penetrating keratoplasty
PP—pressure patch
PRP—panretinal photocoagulation
R&R—resection & recession
RK—radial keratotomy
SB—scleral buckle
SI—sector iridectomy
Vx—vitrectomy

Medicinal/Prescriptions

Units of Measure

cc—cubic centimeters
gm—gram
IU—international units
mg—milligrams
ml—milliliters
mm—millimeters
oz—ounces
tbs—tablespoon
tsp—teaspoon

Forms

cap—capsule
gt—drop
gtt—drops
liq—liquid
tab—tablet
ung—ointment

Directions

i—one
ii—two
iii—three

P/O—by mouth
NPO—without food
a.c.—before meals
p.c.—after meals
i.c.—between meals
a.m.—morning
p.m.—afternoon
d—day
h—hour
p̄—after
q̄—every
qd—every day
bid—twice daily
tid—three times daily
qid—four times daily
qod—every other day
q4h—every 4 hours
hs—bedtime
ut—as directed
prn—as needed
no., # —number
non rep—do not refill
DC—discontinue

Medical Tests

BP—blood pressure
BUN—blood urea nitrogen
CAT—computerized axial tomography
CBC—complete blood count
CT—computerized tomography
ECG/EKG—electrocardia
EUA—evaluation under anesthesia
FBS—fasting blood sugar
GTT—glucose tolerance test
HLA—human leukocyte antigens
MRI—magnetic resonance imaging
RBC—red blood cells
UA—urinalysis
VDRL—syphilis test
WBC—white blood cells

Chemicals/Drugs

ACTH—adrenocorticotropic hormone
ASA—aspirin
BCP—birth control pills
Ca—calcium
DFP—di-isopropyl fluorophosphate (isoflurophate)
EDTA—ethelenediaminotetraacetate sodium
Fe—iron
HCT or HCTZ—hydrochlorothiazide
HRT—hormone replacement therapy
IDU—idoxuridine
K—potassium
Na—sodium
NS—normal saline
O_2—oxygen
PI—phospholine iodide

Miscellaneous

~—approximately
@—at
ant—anterior
ASAP—as soon as possible
ER—emergency room
gen—general
GP—general practitioner
hyper—over
hypo—under
IM—intramuscular
inf—inferior
IV—intravenous
LMD—local medical doctor
max—maximum
min—minimum
neg—negative
norm—normal
OR—operating room
path—pathology
pos—positive
preop—preoperative
prep—prepare
reg—regular

post—posterior
postop—postoperative
prosth—prosthesis
STAT—at once
sup—superior
WCB—will call back

Sample History Using Abbreviations

35 yo wf c/o OD hurting (stabbing pain) X 1-2 wk. Awakens ~2 am qd w/pain. Saw her LMD 5 d ago, who Rx'd gentamicin gtt. Gtt help briefly when eye is hurting, put problem has not DC'd. No discharge, no redness, no ↓ VA. Doesn't really bother her during the day. Pt wears DWDSCL's; never sleeps in them. Cleans w/Renu. No recent solution Δ. Replaces lenses q 3 wk. Has worn this pair X 2 d. Δing lenses hasn't improved pain. No recent ocular injury. POH includes K abr 2° hit in OD by bush, ~2 yr ago.

Translation (*with explained terms underlined*): Thirty-five-year-old white female complains of right eye hurting (stabbing pain) for 1 to 2 weeks. Awakens at approximately 2 in the morning every day with pain. Saw her local medical doctor 5 days ago, who prescribed gentamicin drops. Drops help briefly when eye is hurting, put problem has not discontinued. No discharge, no redness, no decreased vision. Doesn't really bother her during the day. Patient wears daily wear disposable soft contact lenses; never sleeps in them. Cleans with Renu. No recent solution change. Replaces lenses every 3 weeks. Has worn this pair for 2 days. Changing lenses hasn't improved pain. No recent ocular injury. Past ocular history includes corneal abrasion secondary to being hit in the right eye by bush, approximately 2 years ago.

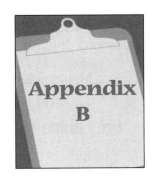

Appendix
B

Appendix B
Spelling and Reference
Guide for Common Drugs
······························

Systemic and Other Non-Ophthalmic Drugs

Note: Most of the drugs in this section were taken from the list of top 200 prescribed drugs of 1996 as cataloged by National Prescription Audit Plus, IMS America, Ltd. All names that start with a capital letter are trade/brand names. Abbreviations are explained folowing the table.

Drug name	Use	Common Brands
Accupril	htn	
Accutane	acne	
acetaminophen	pain	
acetazolamide	glaucoma	Diamox
acyclovir	antiviral	Zovirax
Adalat	htn	
Aerobid	asthma	
albuterol	asthma	Proventil, Ventolin
allopurinol	gout	Zyloprim
alprazolam	anxiety	Xanax
Altace	htn	
Alupent	asthma	
Ambien	sleep	
amitriptyline	antidep, chronic pain	Elavil, Limbitrol
amoxicillin	antibx	Amoxil
Antivert	dizziness	
atenolol	htn	Tenoretic, Tenormin
Atrovent	asthma	
Augmentin	antibx	
Axid	reflux	
Azmacort	asthma	
Bactrim	antibx	
Beconase	allergy	
Benadryl	allergy	
Benemid	gout	
Biaxin	antibx	
Bumex	edema	
BuSpar	anxiety	
captopril	htn	Capoten, Capozide
Carafate	duodenal ulcer	
Cardizem	htn	
Cardura	htn	
Carisoprodol	muscle spasm	Soma

Drug name	Use	Common Brands
Cataflam	anti-infl (NSAID)	
cefaclor	antibx	Ceclor
Ceftin	antibx	
Cefzil	antibx	
cephalexin	antibx	Keflex, Biocef
chloroquine	malaria	
cimetidine	ulcer, reflux	Tagamet
Cipro	antibx	
Claritin	allergies	
Claritin D	nasal cong	
Clinoril	anti-infl (NSAID)	
clonidine	htn	Catapres, Combipres
Clozaril	antipsychotic	
codeine	pain	
Cogentin	Parkinson's	
Cordarone	heart regulator	
Coumadin	anticoag	
Cozaar	htn	
cyclobenzaprine	muscle spasm	Flexeril
Dalmane	insomnia	
Darvocet-N	pain	
Daypro	anti-infl (NSAID)	
Depakote	seizures	
Desogen	BCP	
Diabinese	NIDDM	
diazepam	anxiety	Valium
diclofenac	anti-infl	Voltaren
dicyclomine	GI anti-sps	Bentyl
Diflucan	anti-yeast	
digoxin	heart regulator	Lanoxin
Dilacor	htn	
Dilaudid	pain	
dipyridamole	platelet inhibitor	Persantine
Dolobid	anti-infl (NSAID)	
Donnatal	IBS	
Duricef	antibx	
Effexor	antidepressant	
Entex	nasal cong	
Ery-Tab	antibx	
erythromycin	antibx	
Estrace	HRT	

Drug name	Use	Common Brands
Estraderm	HRT	
Estratest	HRT	
Famvir	antiviral	
Feldene	RA	
Fiorinal	headache	
Flonase	nasal cong	
Floxin	antibx	
Fosamax	osteo	
furosemide	htn/CHF	Lasix
gemfibrozil	cholesterol	Lopid
glipizide	NIDDM	Glucotrol
Glucophage	NIDDM	
glyburide	NIDDM	DiaBeta,Glynase, Micronase
guaifenesin	cough	added to many cold preps
Halcion	insomnia	
Hismanal	allergy	
Hydergine	senile dementia	
Hytrin	htn	
ibuprofen	pain	Motrin, Ibu
Imdur	angina	
Imitrex	migraine	
Imodium	diarrhea	
Inderal	htn, angina	
Indocin	RA	
insulin	IDDM	Humulin,Iletin, Novolin, NPH, Lente
Ismo	angina	
Isordil	angina	
K-Dur	potassium	
Klonopin	seizures	
Klor-Con	potassium	
Lescol	cholesterol	
Levoxyl	hypothyroid	
Levsin	ulcer	
Librax	IBS	
Lo/Ovral	BCP	
Lodine	anti-infl (NSAID)	
Loestrin-FE	BCP	
Lomotil	diarrhea	
Lorabid	antibx	

Drug name	Use	Common Brands
lorazepam	anxiety	Ativan
Lozol	htn/edema	
Ludiomil	antidep	
Macrobid	UTI	
Macrodantin	antibx/UTI	
Maxair	asthma	
medroxy-progesterone	HRT	Amen, Depo-Provera, Prempro, Provera
Mellaril	psychotic disorders	
methyldopa	htn	Aldomet
methylphenidate	ADD	Ritalin
methyl-prednisolone	anti-infl (steroid)	
metoprolol	htn	Lopressor
Mevacor	cholesterol	
Minipress	htn	
Minizide	htn	
Monopril	htn	
naproxen	pain, anti-infl	Aleve, Anaprox, Naprosyn
Neptazane	glaucoma	
Nitro-Dur	angina	
Nitrostat	angina	
Norpace	arrhythmia	
Norvasc	htn	
Ogen	HRT	
Oretic	htn	
Ortho-Cept	BCP	
Ortho-Cyclen	BCP	
Ortho-Novum	BCP	
Ortho-Tri-Cyclen	BCP	
Orudis	anti-infl (NSAID)	
Oruvail	anti-infl (NSAID)	
Pamelor	antidep	
Paxil	depression	
penicillin	antibx	Bicillin, Pen-Vee K, Wycillin
Pepcid	reflux/ulcer	
Percocet	pain	
Percodan	pain	
Perdiem	laxative	
Phenergan	nausea	

Drug name	Use	Common Brands
phenobarbital	sedative	
phentermine	appetite sup	Fastin, Obenix, Zantryl
phenytoin	seizures	Dilantin
Pondimin	appetite sup	
potassium chloride	potassium	
Pravachol	cholesterol	
prednisone	anti-infl (steroid)	Sterapred
Premarin	HRT	
Prevacid	reflux/ulcer	
Prilosec	reflux/ulcer	
Prinivil	htn	
Procardia	htn	
Propacet	pain	
propoxyphene	pain	Darvon
Propulsid	reflux	
Proscar	BPH	
Prozac	depression	
Pyridium	pain of UTI	
Questran	cholesterol	
Quinaglute	heart flutters	
Reglan	reflux	
Relafen	anti-infl (NSAID)	
reserpine	htn	Diupres, Hydropres, Ser-Ap-Es
Retin-A	acne	
Retrovir	HIV	
Risperdal	antipsychotic	
Roxicet	pain	
Salutensin	htn	
Seldane	allergy	
Septra	UTI	
Serevent	asthma/COPD	
Sinemet	Parkinsonism	
Sinequan	depression	
Slo-Bid	asthma, emphysema	
Stelazine	psychotic disorders	
Sudafed	nasal cong	
Suprax	antibx	
Synthroid	hypothyroid	
tamoxifen	cancer	Nolvadex
Tegretol	seizures	

Drug name	Use	Common Brands
temazepam	anxiety	Restoril
Theo-Dur	asthma/COPD	
Thorazine	sedative	
Tofranil	depression	
Tolectin	RA, osteo	
Toprol-XL	htn	
Tranxene	anxiety	
Trental	anti-coag	
Tri-Levlen	BCP	
triamterene	htn	Dyazide
Triavil	anxiety	
trimethoprim	antibx	
Trimox	antibx	
Triphasil	BCP	
Ultram	pain	
Ultrase	pancreatic insufficiency	
Vancenase	nasal cong	
Vanceril	asthma/COPD	
Vasotec	htn	
Veetids	antibx	
verapamil	htn	Calan, Isoptin, Verelan
Vibramycin	antibx	
Vicodin	pain	
Vistaril	anxiety	
Wellbutrin	depression	
Wytensin	htn	
Zantac	reflux/ulcer	
Zestoretic	htn	
Zestril	htn	
Zithromax	antibx	
Zocor	cholesterol	
Zoloft	depression	
Zyrtec	allergy	

Abbreviations:

ADD—attention deficit disorder
antibx—antibiotic
anticoag—anticoagulant
antidep—antidepressant
anti-infl—anti-inflammatory
antisps—antispasmodic

BCP—birth control pills
BPH—benign prostatic hyperplasia
CHF—congestive heart failure
cong—congestion
COPD—chronic obstructive pulmonary disease
GI—gastrointestinal
HIV—human immunodeficiency virus
HRT—hormone replacement therapy
Htn—anti-hypertensive
IBS—irritable bowel syndrome
IDDM—insulin-dependent diabetes mellitus
NIDDM—non-insulin-dependent diabetes mellitus
NSAID—nonsteroidal anti-inflammatory drug
osteo—osteoporosis
RA—rheumatoid arthritis
reflux refers to esophageal reflux
sup—suppressant
ulcer refers to gastric ulcer (unless otherwise noted)
UTI—urinary tract infection

Common Ophthalmic Drugs

All drugs listed are brand names, which are registered trademarks.

Acular	anti-infl (NSAID)
AK-Cide	antibx/steroid (sulfa)
AK-Dex	anti-infl (steroid)
AK-Poly-Bac	antibx (combo)
AK-Trol	antibx/steroid
Albalon	decong
Alphagan-P	glaucoma
Aquify	dry eye
Betagan	glaucoma
Betimol	glaucoma
Betoptic	glaucoma
Bion Tears	dry eye
Bleph 10	antibx (sulfa)
Bleph 30	antibx (sulfa)
Blephamide	antibx/steroid (sulfa)
Carboptic	glaucoma
Celluvisc	dry eye
Ciloxan	antibx
Collyrium Fresh	decong

Cortisporin	antibx/steroid
CoSopt	glaucoma
Crolom	mast cell stabilizer
Dendrid	antiviral
Dexacine	antibx/steroid
E-Pilo	glaucoma
Econopred Plus	anti-infl (steroid)
Elestat	antihis
Epifrin	glaucoma
Flarex	anti-infl (steroid)
Flour-op	anti-infl (steroid)
FML	anti-infl (steroid)
FML-S	antibx/steroid (sulfa)
Genoptic	antibx
Gentak	antibx
GenTeal	dry eye
Glaucon	glaucoma
HMS	anti-infl (steroid)
homatropine	cycloplegia
HypoTears	dry eye
Inflamase	anti-infl (steroid)
Iopidine	glaucoma
Isopto Carbachol	glaucoma
Isopto Carpine	glaucoma
Isopto Cetamide	antibx (sulfa)
Lacrilube	dry eye
Lacrisert	dry eye
Maxidex	anti-infl (steroid)
Maxitrol	antibx/steroid
Murine Plus	decong
Muro 128	corneal edema
Naphcon	decong
Naphcon-A	decong/antihs
Natacyn	antifungal
NeoDecadron	antibx/steroid
Neosporin	antibx (combo)
OcuClear	decong
Ocucoat	dry eye
Ocufen	anti-infl (NSAID)
Ocuflox	antibx
OcuHist	decong/antihs
Ocupress	glaucoma
Ocusulf	antibx (sulfa)

OptiPranolol	glaucoma
Patanol	antihis
Phospholine Iodide	glaucoma
Pilocar	glaucoma
Pilopine	glaucoma
Poly-Pred	antibx/steroid
Polysporin	antibx (combo)
Polytrim	antibx (combo)
Pred Forte	anti-infl (steroid)
Pred-G	antibx/steroid
Propine	glaucoma
Refresh	dry eye
Restasis	dry eye
Sodium Sulamyd	antibx (sulfa)
Sulf-10	antibx (sulfa)
Sulfamide	antibx/steroid (sulfa)
Systane	dry eye
Tears Naturale	dry eye
Timoptic	glaucoma
TobraDex	antibx/steroid
Tobrex	antibx
Travatan	glaucoma
Trusopt	glaucoma
Ultratears	dry eye
Vasocidin	antibx/steroid (sulfa)
Vasoclear	decong
Vasocon	decong
Vasocon-A	decong/antihs
Vexol	anti-infl (steroid)
Vigamox	antibx
Viroptic	antiviral
Visine AC	decong/astr
Visine LR	decong
Visine	decong
Voltaren	anti-infl (NSAID)
Xalatan	glaucoma
Zaditor	mast cell stabilizer

Abbreviations

antibx—antibiotic
antihs—antihistamine
anti-infl—anti-inflammatory
astr—astringent
combo—combination
decong—decongestant
NSAID—nonsteriodal anti-inflammatory drug

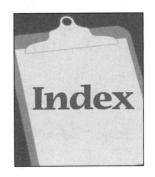

Index
●●●●●●●●●●●●●●●●●●●●●●●●●●●

Index

For your information

This book and many others on numerous different topics are available from SLACK Incorporated. For further information or a copy of our latest catalog, contact us at:

Professional Book Division
SLACK Incorporated
6900 Grove Road
Thorofare, NJ 08086 USA
Telephone: 1-609-848-1000
1-800-257-8290
Fax: 1-609-853-5991
E-mail: orders@slackinc.com
WWW: http://www.slackinc.com

We accept most major credit cards and checks or money orders in US dollars drawn on a US bank. Most orders are shipped within 72 hours.

Contact us for information on recent releases, forthcoming titles, and bestsellers. If you have a comment about this title or see a need for a new book, direct your correspondence to the Editorial Director at the above address.

If you are an instructor, we can be reached at the address listed above or on the Internet at **educomps@slackinc.com** *for specific needs.*

Thank you for your interest and we hope you found this work beneficial.